COMMISSIONING FOR HEALTH AND WELL-BEING

An introduction

Edited by Jon Glasby

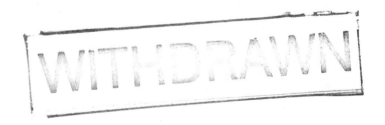

First published in Great Britain in 2012 by

The Policy Press
University of Bristol
Fourth Floor
Beacon House
Queen's Road
Bristol BS8 1QU, UK
t: +44 (0)117 331 4054
f: +44 (0)117 331 4093
tpp-info@bristol.ac.uk
www.policypress.co.uk

North American office:
The Policy Press
c/o The University of Chicago Press
1427 East 60th Street
Chicago, IL 60637, USA
t: +1 773 702 7700
f: +1 773-702-9756
sales@press.uchicago.edu
www.press.uchicago.edu

© The Policy Press 2012

British Library Cataloguing in Publication Data
A catalogue record for this book is available from the British Library.

Library of Congress Cataloging-in-Publication Data
A catalog record for this book has been requested.

ISBN 978 1 84742 792 2 paperback
ISBN 978 1 84742 793 9 hardcover

The right of Jon Glasby to be identified as editor of this work has been asserted by him in accordance with the Copyright, Designs and Patents Act 1988.

The Policy Press uses environmentally responsible print partners.

Cover design by Qube Design Associates, Bristol
Front cover: photograph kindly supplied by istock.com
Printed and bound in Great Britain by Hobbs, Southampton

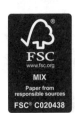

Contents

List of boxes, figures and tables

Boxes

Figures

Tables

List of abbreviations

Although not exhaustive, the list below sets out some of the key/common abbreviations used in this book and in broader debates about commissioning. While the technical terms often remain the same, some of the names of government departments may change over time and some may be listed here under a historical name if they have been subject to previous or recent rebranding.

A4R	Accountability for Reasonableness
ADASS	Association of Directors of Adult Social Services
ADLAY	activity of daily living adjusted year
BHLP	budget-holding lead professional
BSF	Building Schools for the Future
CAMHS	childhood and adolescent mental health services
CBA	cost-benefit analysis
CBI	Confederation of British Industry
CCT	compulsory competitive tendering
CEA	cost-effectiveness analysis
CIPFA	Chartered Institute of Public Finance and Accountancy
CQUIN	Commissioning for Quality and Innovation
CRD	Centre for Reviews and Dissemination
CUA	cost-utility analysis
DCLG	Department for Communities and Local Government
DCSF	Department for Children, Schools and Families
DEFRA	Department for Environment, Food and Rural Affairs
DH	Department of Health
DWP	Department for Work and Pensions
EU	European Union
GDP	Gross Domestic Product
GP	general practitioner
HEED	Health Economics Evaluations Database
HMSO/TSO	Her Majesty's Stationery Office/The Stationery Office
HSMC	Health Services Management Centre
HTA	Health Technology Assessment
ICER	Incremental Cost-Effectiveness Ratio
ICT	information and communication technology
INLOGOV	Institute of Local Government Studies
JSNA	Joint Strategic Needs Assessment
LAA	Local Area Agreement
LGA	Local Government Association
LIFT	Local Infrastructure Finance Trust
LSP	local strategic partnership

MMDM	MASLIN Multi-Dimensional Matrix
NAO	National Audit Office
NHS	National Health Service
NICE	National Institute for Health and Clinical Excellence
NPM	New Public Management
OECD	Organisation for Economic Co-operation and Development
ONS	Office for National Statistics
OPM	Office for Public Management
OTS	Office of the Third Sector
PALS	Patient Advocacy and Liaison Service
PBMA	programme budgeting and marginal analysis
PCT	primary care trust
PFI	Private Finance Initiative
PPI	public and patient involvement
PSSRU	Personal Social Services Research Unit
QALY	quality-adjusted life year
QOF	Quality and Outcomes Framework
RAS	resource allocation system
SCIE	Social Care Institute for Excellence
SIGN	Scottish Intercollegiate Guidelines Network
SPRU	Social Policy Research Unit
SRM	supplier relationship management
TCE	transaction cost economics
TUPE	Transfer of Undertakings (Protection of Employment) Regulations
UK	United Kingdom
US	United States
VBP	value-based purchasing
VFM	value for money
YOT	Youth Offending Team

Notes on contributors

Kerry Allen is a research fellow at the University of Birmingham's Health Services Management Centre (HSMC), with an interest in joint working, disability and community care.

Tony Bovaird is Professor of Public Management and Policy at the Institute of Local Government Studies (INLOGOV), University of Birmingham, with an interest in performance management in the public sector and the strategic management of public organisations.

Helen Dickinson is a senior lecturer at HSMC, with an interest in health and social partnerships, leadership and the role of the third sector.

Simon Duffy is an honorary senior fellow at HSMC and Director of The Centre for Welfare Reform, with an interest in personalisation, citizenship and the transformation of public services.

Jo Ellins is a lecturer at HSMC, with an interest in public and patient engagement in health and social care.

Jon Glasby is Director of HSMC and Professor of Health and Social Care, with an interest in joint working between health and social care, community care services and personalisation.

Eleanor Hothersall is a clinical lecturer in public health at the University of Birmingham, with an interest in chronic obstructive pulmonary disease, and physical activity and the built environment.

Chris Lonsdale is a senior lecturer and Head of the Procurement and Operations Management Group at the Birmingham Business School, with an interest in outsourcing, public–private partnerships and purchaser–supplier relationships.

Tom Marshall is a senior lecturer at the School of Health and Population Sciences, University of Birmingham, with an interest in needs assessment, quality improvement and primary care services.

Catherine Needham is a senior lecturer at Queen Mary, University of London, and writes on public policy reform and political communication.

Alyson Nicholds is a research fellow at HSMC, undertaking national research around the outcomes of joint commissioning.

Lesley Prince, formerly Lecturer in Organisational Behaviour at the Institute of Local Government Studies, University of Birmingham and Visiting Lecturer at Warwick Business School, is now a freelance academic social psychologist with extensive experience working in and with public sector, private sector and third sector organisations on organisational behaviour issues.

Ray Puffitt is an honorary senior lecturer at INLOGOV, with an interest in local government management, performance management and commissioning and contracting.

Suzanne Robinson is a lecturer at HSMC, with an interest in decision making and priority setting, strategic commissioning and health economics.

Iestyn Williams is a lecturer at HSMC, with an interest in decision making and priority setting, public value and the spread of innovation.

Peter Watt is a reader in public sector economics at INLOGOV, specialising in local government finance, the economics of procurement and contracting, and public sector efficiency.

Martin Willis is an honorary senior lecturer at INLOGOV, with an interest in strategic commissioning, outcomes-based approaches and service user involvement.

Acknowledgements

All the authors of this edited collection are based at or associated with the University of Birmingham – and are grateful to current and previous students on the university's various commissioning-related MScs, CPD programmes, workshops and learning sets. This book has very much arisen out of our research, teaching, consultancy and policy advice in the National Health Service and local government, and we are grateful to colleagues from policy and practice for their help in developing our ideas and key frameworks.

We are also grateful to The Policy Press for all their help and support.

Note: Discussions of the impact of commissioning-led approaches to health and social care in the Introduction to this book draw heavily on previous analysis conducted by Jon Glasby, Chris Ham and colleagues for a Department of Health/Downing Street-funded review of adult social care costs and reform (Glasby et al, 2010), and some of this text is reproduced in the Introduction to the current book with the permission of Professor Chris Ham (the main author of the relevant section of the report).

See: Glasby, J., Ham, C., Littlechild, R. and McKay, S. (2010) *The case for social care reform: The wider economic and social benefits* (for the Department of Health/Downing Street), Birmingham: HSMC/Institute of Applied Social Studies.

At the time of writing, all government departments and web addresses were correct – although the new government was in the process of archiving previous material and changing the layout and focus of some departmental websites.

Introduction

Jon Glasby

Summary

This chapter explores:
- the aims and scope of the book;
- key definitions;
- the origins, nature and impact of commissioning;
- key rationales for a commissioning-led approach.

Although only 'quick and dirty', it is still revealing to enter 'commissioning' as a search term via Google. In 2009, there were some 835,000 UK entries for 'commissioning + Department of Health' – compared to 356,000 in 1999 and 220,000 in 1989. While this is partly to do with the changing role of the internet, it also suggests a potentially dramatic increase in official use of the term 'commissioning'. Thus, recent years have seen the publication of a plethora of health and social care policy documents with commissioning as a key focus – including a 'world class commissioning' agenda for the National Health Service (NHS), a commitment to (general practitioner: GP) 'practice-based commissioning', guidance on 'commissioning for health and well-being', increasing emphasis on 'joint commissioning', growing discussion of 'total place' commissioning, a 'strategic commissioning' agenda across broader local government and a firm commitment to 'commissioning for personalisation' in adult social care. The latest version following a 2010 White Paper (DH, 2010a) is 'GP commissioning consortia'. All this raises a series of key questions:

- What is commissioning?
- Why does it matter?
- Where has it come from?
- What has it achieved?
- What does this mean in practice?
- Where might it take us?

Of course, previous policy in both health and social care has tended to identify specific individuals or organisations primarily responsible for deciding what services are needed and making sure that they are provided (often described as 'purchasing') and those who actually deliver such services (the 'providers'). While this is a longstanding distinction, there have been a number of key changes:

- First of all, early policy in the later 1980s and early 1990s often encouraged 'purchasers' to 'buy' services from public sector providers (a form of 'internal market' rather than a genuinely open market where purchasers can choose services from any willing provider from the public, private or voluntary sector) – particularly in the NHS.
- Over time, this has begun to shift with – rhetorically at least – a much more mixed economy of service providers (and in some areas of policy a range of new service providers from the private and voluntary sectors competing on more of a level playing field, with increasingly arm's-length or separate public sector providers).
- In some cases, this has led to the growth of new, hybrid organisational forms, crossing traditional divides between public, private and voluntary sectors. Examples here might include social enterprises, NHS foundation trusts or maybe even employee-owned organisations.
- There has been a shift away from simply purchasing various back-office or infrastructure services externally towards purchasing a broader range of people-focused health and social care services (including clinical services).
- There has been a broadening of the focus from simply 'purchasing' externally to a more all-encompassing notion of 'commissioning' (see below for further discussion of key definitions).
- There has been a recognition of the need to move away from a single agency focus towards a more inter-agency or even whole-system approach.
- Finally, there has been a greater awareness of the need to commission different services at different levels, including at the level of individual service users, patients and citizens where appropriate.

However, perhaps the most significant shift has been a transition from organisations that combine purchasing and provision, towards a situation where health (and to some extent social care) agencies are increasingly expected to *primarily* (or even *only*) commission – 'steering, not rowing' as it is often described. A good example of this is the previous NHS world class commissioning agenda, which forced the rapid evolution of primary care trusts (PCTs) away from organisations that combined the commissioning of acute care with the provision of community health services, to new entities (possibly merging to become larger in future), which were entirely (or almost entirely) focused on commissioning. As a result, community health services were floated off as stand-alone entities (perhaps as social enterprises or community foundation trusts), integrated with acute or mental health trusts and/or integrated with local government. Arguably, this made the role of PCTs very different to the way in which they operated in the past, requiring different skills, behaviours and approaches. Although health policy is changing rapidly at the time of writing, such issues will be just as relevant for new GP consortia.

Audience and content

Against this background, there is an urgent need for more detailed and focused development opportunities to equip health and social care commissioners to meet such a challenging and fundamental agenda. Although commissioning is currently a key priority, many commentators would argue that the policy context has evolved so rapidly that we still lack a sufficient infrastructure to make a reality of recent commitments to a commissioning-led approach. If we are serious about commissioning being the answer to a range of current challenges in both health and social care, then how are we going to make commissioning the career of choice for future NHS and local government leaders? Where are the commissioning-focused MScs, MBAs and development programmes? Where is the Royal College of Health and Social Care Commissioners? Without these things, surely there is a danger that commissioning is simply set up to fail, floundering under the weight of unrealistic expectation without being given the tools to really deliver. While this has always been true, current funding cuts, the rapid extension of personalisation and the development of GP-led commissioning all make these issues even more topical.

In response to this agenda, the University of Birmingham (with which the current authors are all associated) has become one of the leading providers of commissioning-related training and development opportunities for health and social care managers and clinicians. Over time this has included a number of MSc programmes in Healthcare Commissioning for various strategic health authorities, a PG Certificate for the Welsh National Leadership and Innovation Agency for Health and an MSc believed to be the first programme of its kind in the United Kingdom (UK) for NHS and local government managers interested in cross-public service commissioning. Throughout this process, a common concern from participants is that they have been unable to find a basic introductory textbook to gain a rapid overview of some of the key issues, with the policy context feeling as if it is some way ahead of current research, teaching and academic publications. While there have been some key contributions to date (see the end of this chapter for further reading), this does seem indicative of the rapidly evolving nature of the policy context. Hardly surprisingly, it is this gap that the current textbook aims to fill – and we believe that this may be the first UK textbook of its kind.

Building on Birmingham's reputation in this important area of policy and practice, all the contributors to this edited collection are based at or linked with the University of Birmingham, from the Health Services Management Centre (HSMC), the Institute of Local Government Studies (INLOGOV), the Birmingham Business School and the Public Health Unit. Above all, this book is intended to be an introductory textbook for health and social care managers and policy makers, as well as for students of public policy. With the advent of GP commissioning consortia, moreover, we hope that the book will be relevant to the growing number of clinicians involved in commissioning and in management roles more generally. It explores a range of issues, including:

- the policy context and political environment in which strategic commissioning has become a core element of public service management;
- how commissioning and procurement have emerged in the context of wider public sector reform, and how they might develop in future;
- some of the key theoretical models underpinning public service commissioning;
- the economics of commissioning (and decommissioning);
- different approaches to decision making and priority setting in the allocation of public resources;
- different approaches to and the impact of involving the public in strategic commissioning;
- commissioning in an era of personalisation;
- commissioning for quality and outcomes.

Throughout, the focus is both on health and social care commissioning and on applying lessons from research and theory to policy and practice. As a result, we have chosen to include a range of different contributors who bring different perspectives from across the NHS and local government, from the independent sector, from theory and applied research, and from policy and management. Although individual topics and writing styles inevitably vary, we have tried to provide a degree of continuity, with each chapter including a summary of the key issues covered; a review of key themes and issues; further reading and useful websites; and reflective exercises for health and social care practitioners, managers and policy makers. Alongside this collection, a number of the key themes below are explored in more detail in a second book by Williams et al (2011) entitled *Rationing in health care: the theory and practice of priority setting*.

As an introduction to the book, this chapter offers some brief definitions, provides an overview of the emergence of commissioning as a key activity of local public services, reviews the evidence (and often the lack of evidence) behind the strategic commissioning agenda and explores the rationales behind these changes. Next, Part One of the book focuses on different aspects of the commissioning cycle. In Chapter One, Tony Bovaird, Helen Dickinson and Kerry Allen review the different models of commissioning emerging across different government departments, considering their strengths and limitations, the contexts in which they are likely to be appropriate and the situations where they are less likely to work. In Chapter Two, Tom Marshall and Eleanor Hothersall focus on the issue of needs, demand and supply, which includes a discussion of different underlying approaches to needs assessment and some of the practical tools and techniques available. In Chapter Three, Iestyn Williams and Suzanne Robinson explore the priority-setting process, considering the political and ethical elements of commissioning as well as some of the more technical economic and epidemiological perspectives. This is followed by Chris Lonsdale's summary of the key principles of effective procurement (Chapter Four), drawing on insights from the commercial sector and stressing the need to understand relationships with providers as involving elements of both cooperation and competition. This is followed by two contributions by Ray Puffitt and Lesley Prince (Chapters Five and Six) on the often-neglected topics of decommissioning and of commissioning for service resilience in the face of economic dislocation. Finally in Part One, Martin Willis and Tony Bovaird focus on the crucial issue of commissioning for quality and for outcomes (Chapter Seven), exploring how this works in practice, its strengths and its limitations.

In Part Two of the book, four chapters focus on a number of cross-cutting, underlying themes. In Chapter Eight, Peter Watt sets out the key economic principles that are important in commissioning services, discussing issues such as incentives, information and trust. Next, Jo Ellins explores the issue of public and user involvement in the commissioning cycle (Chapter Nine), summarising the policy context and providing a critical review of progress to date. This is followed in Chapter Ten by Helen Dickinson and Alyson Nicholds' discussion of joint commissioning, exploring the extent to which more joined-up approaches have genuinely led to different and better outcomes for people using services. Building on similar themes, Catherine Needham and Simon Duffy examine the implications of the current personalisation agenda in health and social care (Chapter Eleven), reviewing recent progress as well as outlining key challenges for the future.

In Part Three of the book, a short conclusion pulls together key themes and sets out some implications for future policy, practice and research (Chapter Twelve).

What is commissioning and why does it matter?

According to the Department of Health (2010b), 'Commissioning in the NHS is the process of ensuring that the health and care services provided effectively meet the needs of the population. It is a complex process with responsibilities ranging from assessing population needs, prioritising health outcomes, procuring products and services, and managing service providers.' Typically, this is depicted as a cycle, in which health and social care organisations assess needs, plan services, contract with providers, monitor quality and outcomes and revise accordingly. Building on such approaches and definitions, Woodin (2006, p 203) argues that:

> Commissioning ... tends to denote a proactive strategic role in planning, designing and implementing the range of services required, rather than a more passive purchasing role. A commissioner decides which services or ... interventions should be provided, who should provide them, and how they should be paid for, and may work closely with the provider in implementing changes.

These definitions are helpful up to a point (especially the work of Woodin – see Box i.1), but the official descriptions in particular tend to be so broad that it can be difficult to drill down to pinpoint some of the key details (see also Chapter One by Bovaird et al). However, to flesh this out Wade et al (2006, p 5) draw on the work of Smith and Mays (2005) to portray commissioning as the 'brain', the 'conscience' and the 'eyes and ears' of the system. Thus, the key roles of health and social care commissioners are:

- Conscience – setting out 'how things should be' – what the system aims to achieve and how.
- Eyes and ears – observing and reporting on 'how things are' – what the system is currently delivering.
- Brain (having processed information from both sources) – identifying and implementing the optimal solutions for delivering stated objectives. (Wade et al, 2006, p 3)

Over time, managers in health and social care commissioning roles have repeatedly fed back how helpful they find this analogy. While 'brain' and 'eyes and ears' functions appear in official commissioning cycles, it is often the notion of commissioning as the 'conscience' of the local system that resonates most.

Box i.1: Key definitions

Commissioning is 'the set of linked activities required to assess the ... needs of a population, specify the services required to meet those needs within a strategic framework, secure those services, monitor and evaluate the outcomes'.

Purchasing is 'the process of buying or funding services in response to demand or usage'.

Contracting is 'the technical process of selecting a provider, negotiating and agreeing the terms of a contract for services, and ongoing management of the contract including payment, monitoring, variations'.

Procurement is 'the process of identifying a supplier, and may involve for example competitive tendering, competitive quotation, single sourcing. It may also involve stimulating the market through awareness raising and education'.

Source: Woodin (2006, p 204), Wade et al (2006, p 3)

Moving beyond issues of definition, a number of policy documents and other commentators set out a list of the key things that a commissioning-led approach is meant to achieve. For the Department of Health (DH, 2007), for example, commissioning can be a tool in order to achieve:

- better health and well-being for all (with people living healthier and longer lives and with health inequalities being dramatically reduced);

- better care for all (with services that are evidence based and of the best quality, and with people having choice and control over the services that they use, so they become more personalised);
- better value for all (where investment decisions are made in an informed and considered way, ensuring that improvements are delivered within available resources, and where PCTs work with others to optimise effective care).

For Mays and Hand (2000, quoted in Ham, 2008, p 2), commissioning has emerged as a key element of reform in a range of developed countries in order to:

- improve technical efficiency by allowing purchasers to select the best value provider accessible to their populations, including private and voluntary sector providers, thereby giving purchasers some control over providers;
- allow those charged with determining the future pattern of health services in relation to the needs of the population to concentrate on this task unhindered by their previous responsibilities for managing healthcare institutions and, at the same time, allow the providers to manage their own affairs with the minimum of unnecessary interference;
- act as a counterweight to decades of professional dominance of service specification and to challenge traditional patterns of resource allocation and sectional interests (active purchasing rather than passive funding or bureaucratic planning);
- improve allocative efficiency by permitting purchasers to negotiate a new balance of services with providers;
- encourage providers to respond more accurately and effectively to the needs of individual patients in order to retain contracts from purchasers;
- facilitate clear lines of public accountability for the performance of the purchaser and provider roles in the health system;
- clarify providers' costs and the amount spent in each service area by comparing the services and costs of each provider;
- make priority decisions more explicit.

In practice, the extent to which commissioning-led approaches have delivered the aspirations of policy makers remains open to question (see, for example, Mays and Hand, 2000; Ashton et al, 2004; Smith et al, 2004; Figueras et al, 2005; Greve, 2008; Ham, 2008) – see below for further discussion.

Where has commissioning come from?

Public service commissioning has received increasing attention in a number of countries as part of a worldwide process of reform. In this process, governments have separated the provision of public services from commissioning in the belief that this will result in improvements in performance. Reforms based on the commissioner–provider split have been used to introduce greater competition into the provision of public services. This includes encouraging new providers to compete for contracts as services are market tested (see Greve, 2008, for a review of international experience). While the initial interest in introducing competition into the provision of public services was led by governments of the centre-right, this approach has since been taken forward by politicians of different persuasions as the pace of reform has quickened.

Whatever the claims made by policy makers around the practical benefits (or otherwise) of such approaches, most commentators acknowledge that the current emphasis on commissioning is more to do with changing trends within the broader political, economic, social and technological environment. If commissioning has emerged as a key reform mechanism in a range of sectors and in a range of different countries at the same time, it is likely to be because there are broader changes under way. In particular, the current emphasis on commissioning-led approaches can be seen as a response to the development of New Public Management (NPM) – a series of public sector reforms based essentially around the incorporation of perceived best practice from the private sector into traditional public services (see, for example, McLaughlin et al, 2002). Driven by rising public expectations, changing demography, technological advances and the economic crises of the late 1970s, a range of governments began to initiate reforms based on a move away from 'traditional' public administration towards new approaches, borrowing more commercial concepts and processes such as:

- setting and measuring clear objectives and outcomes;
- disaggregating traditional bureaucracies and decentralising authority (but holding the front line more to account for performance);
- use of market mechanisms to drive down costs and improve quality;
- placing a greater emphasis on customer responsiveness.

While this process is described in more detail elsewhere (see, for example, McLaughlin et al, 2002; Greve, 2008), the current commissioning agenda should be seen not so much as a stand-alone policy from a government keen to reform health and social care, but as a response to a broader series of changes in how public services are conceived, managed and delivered.

Against this background, a helpful framework is provided by Julian Le Grand (2003, 2007), a leading social policy academic and a former health adviser to Tony Blair. According to Le Grand, public services can be organised and reformed in at least four different ways:

- *trust* – trusting frontline services and professions to do a good job in the interests of their service users;
- *targets* – a form of command and control, with rewards or penalties for hitting specific (often numerical) targets;
- *voice* – scope for people using services to express any dissatisfaction with providers;

- *choice and competition* – greater competition between different service providers and choice between these providers by people using the services concerned.

While arguing that each of these mechanisms has strengths and limitations (and that each needs to be used together as part of a wider blend of approaches), Le Grand (2007, p 61) is clear that 'a combination of choice and competition can provide the right incentives for providers to deliver a response service of high quality – a service that respects its users and that is produced in an efficient and equitable fashion'. To some extent, therefore, the need to create greater choice and competition (from a situation in which some public sector providers may traditionally have had a virtual monopoly) might be seen as requiring some sort of profession or organisation to manage/oversee such a transition locally and to make sure that such an agenda really works – hence strategic commissioning. As public expectations continue to rise, moreover, there is less and less acceptance of 'one-size-fits-all' approaches and a demand from the public for much more tailored and personalised approaches (see also Chapter Eleven, this volume).

What impact is commissioning having?

Viewing the current commissioning agenda as a product of a series of international trends in public sector reform is a useful start – not least because it may help to explain (at least in part) why commissioning-led approaches have been driven so hard in spite of the ambiguous nature of the evidence base. Within social care, a review of 10 years of social care markets in England (Knapp et al, 2001, p 304) has argued that 'choice, quality and cost effectiveness improvements seem to be following', although no hard evidence is provided to support this statement. The study also draws attention to the challenges involved in developing social care markets, including asymmetry of information between commissioners and providers and the dangers of risk exploitation.

Since this review, there has been surprisingly little systematic research into the performance of social care markets and the impact of commissioning. However, one of the most recent assessments of the experience of local authorities in using competition to improve performance carried out by the Audit Commission (2007) paints a mixed picture. On the one hand, the review found that up to £80 million of efficiency improvements in corporate services could be attributed to the use of market mechanisms. On the other, it highlighted a series of challenges facing local authorities, including lack of sufficient people with procurement, risk or contract management skills, a shortage of information about local public service markets and inexperience in deciding when to use outsourced provision or in-house services. Overall, the Audit Commission recommended adopting a pragmatic mindset and seeking to fill gaps in skills and information in order to use competition and contestability more effectively.

Alongside longstanding experience in local government, the UK also has experience of healthcare commissioning dating back to the internal market reforms of the 1990s. Although local government has in many ways a much longer track record in this area, there is nevertheless a more substantial literature on healthcare commissioning. Thus, one key review of the evidence (Smith et al, 2004, p 2 – emphasis added) found that:

- 'There is little substantive research evidence to demonstrate that any commissioning approach has made a significant or strategic impact on secondary care services
- Primary care-led commissioning (where clinicians have a clear influence over budgets) can however secure improved responsiveness such as shorter waiting times for treatment and more information on patients' progress ...
- Primary care-led commissioning made its greatest impact in primary and intermediate care, for example in developing a wider range of practice-based services ...
- Given a sustained opportunity to innovate, highly determined managers and clinicians are able to use their commissioning role to change longstanding practices in the local health system ...
- Primary care commissioners can effect change in prescribing practice, with financial incentives playing a key role ...
- Primary care-led commissioning increases transaction costs within commissioning.'

The need to make available adequate resources to support healthcare commissioning is a recurring theme in the literature and is underlined by evidence indicating that Total Purchasing Pilots with higher levels of management cost achieved the best outcomes (Mays et al, 2001). The difficulty in acting on this evidence is that recent reforms to the NHS were designed to *reduce* management costs. Of course, these findings are all the more significant given the recent advent of GP-led commissioning and an urgent need to learn from these previous lessons.

Internationally, the most comprehensive study of healthcare commissioning in Europe (Figueras et al, 2005) found that:

- One size of commissioning organisation will not fit all needs, and devolution of decision making has advantages; however, some functions require a national approach (for example public health and equity).
- The appropriate level of commissioning will depend on conditions such as the type of services to be purchased, the incidence and prevalence of different conditions, the number of places where the necessary services can be provided efficiently, and the appropriate size of the risk pool to handle risk.
- Active contracting is a fairly new activity in many countries, having only really developed during the 1990s, and its development is uneven.
- For contracting to work, providers must have management and financial flexibility to respond to the contract's demands and incentives.

• Needs assessment is not routinely carried out in many systems, and when it is it may not be incorporated into commissioning decisions.

Figueras and colleagues emphasised that a central lesson from European experience is that if policy makers are to achieve desired results they need to take a broad systems approach to commissioning and act on all the various components of this function. They particularly stressed the need for commissioners to have the skills to commission care effectively, commenting:

> Overall, the political, technical and financial ability to implement strategic purchasing is the single most important factor in determining its success or otherwise. Most, if not all, strategies reviewed here are very complex and require a high level of technical and managerial skills together with wide ranging information systems that are lacking in many countries. (Figueras et al, 2005, p 7)

These findings are echoed in studies of healthcare commissioning outside Europe (Ashton et al, 2004). For example, a review of experience in New Zealand reported that lack of good information on costs, volumes and quality made it difficult for commissioners to compare providers' performance and negotiate contracts. Together with the legalistic approach taken in New Zealand, this encouraged an adversarial environment. Negotiations were often acrimonious and transaction costs were high. These challenges were compounded by a shortage of skills among commissioners and providers, especially legal expertise and contract negotiation skills. A further consideration was that competition law concerns were at odds with other objectives, making it difficult to develop longer-term contracts or cooperative relationships. The development of these relationships was hindered by repeated structural reorganisations and changes in personnel.

In the United States (US), there has been recent interest in the development of 'value-based purchasing' (VBP), defined as the following:

> The concept of value-based health care purchasing is that buyers should hold providers of health care accountable for both the cost and quality of care. Value-based purchasing brings together information on the quality of health care, including patient outcomes and health status, with data on the dollar outlays going towards health. It focuses on managing the use of the health care system to reduce inappropriate care and to identify and reward best-performing providers. (Silow-Caroll and Alteras, 2007, p 18)

Research into early examples of VBP concluded that it was too early to measure their impact in a quantifiable way. At an anecdotal level, there was evidence of positives, such as health plans and providers using information on comparative performance to improve the quality of care they offered. At the same time, a number of challenges were noted, including getting consumers to use such information. In summary, the authors noted:

> A considerable amount of time must be available for VBP initiatives to gain significant participation and reach the critical mass needed to make an impact on their local market. The case study sites highlighted in this report have a good head start, but replication in other regions that have different histories and cultures may be more challenging. The value-driven health care movement will be further slowed by attempts to address the technical and other formidable challenges described in this report. (Silow-Caroll and Alteras, 2007, p 19)

Further grounds for caution are to be found in a recent analysis of the travails of healthcare in the US by the chair and chief executive officer of the country's largest integrated delivery system. This analysis argues that a fundamental weakness of the healthcare market in the US is the absence of effective buyers:

> Car manufacturers purchase component parts for their cars all the time with a very high level of competency. The specifications for purchasing hubcaps extend to a thousandth, even millionths, of an inch, to the actual molecular composition of the hubcap material, and to error rates and delivery times for the hubcaps production process.... Health care purchasing has not been held to similar standards. But when we have reached the point where the costs of health care at GM [General Motors] exceeds the cost of steel in a car and the cost of health care coverage at Starbucks exceeds the actual cost of coffee, then it's time for the major buyers to stop thinking of health care as a cost-plus, unengineered, externally shaped, seller-defined, completely unmanaged purchasing expense. It's time for buyers to subject health care to the same kind of detailed performance expectations or specifications as they use for their core business products, and to introduce a whole new level of expertise and leverage into the purchase of both health care coverage and health care delivery. (Halvorson, 2007, p 20)

Overall, evidence from different sources underlines the difficulties in commissioning public services, including health and social care. In summary, three points should be emphasised:

- First, as Figueras et al (2005) noted in their review of experience in Europe, the impact of commissioning will be affected not only by the skills and competences of commissioners and the resources available to them, but also by the architecture of the markets that are put in place. This includes how these markets are regulated and the payment systems that are used.

- Second, as Knapp et al (2001) commented in their review of social care markets, there are fundamental questions to be asked about whether the conditions exist for markets to function effectively in complex public services such as health and social care. These conditions include the availability of information to enable commissioners to carry out their functions, and the ability to write service specifications and contracts to avoid provider dominance.
- Finally, the evidence suggests that where progress has been made it is often via large, well-resourced organisations, with very skilled and expert staff. As Light suggests in a US context:

> The best American commissioning groups have concluded that health care is far more complicated to purchase than anything else – mainframe computers, aircraft, telecommunications systems – you name it. Their salary and bonus packages are designed to attract the best and the brightest. They require excellent data system analysts and programmers, clinical epidemiologists, clinical managers, organisational experts, financial specialists and legal advisers. (Light, 1998, p 67, quoted in Ham, 2008, p 4)

Whether such preconditions are likely to exist in a UK health and social care context any time soon – particularly in a period of significant financial restraint – remains to be seen.

Despite these challenging conclusions, the fact remains that health and social care commissioning is the only game in town – and this seems unlikely to change in the short term (in England at least). While policy and management ideas evolve, the current commissioning agenda seems very firmly embedded and public services will continue to have to find ways of responding to changing needs and rising public expectations. Against this background, the challenge for health and social care managers and clinicians is to recognise the complex but fundamental nature of the challenges they face, to develop their knowledge of different aspects of the commissioning cycle, to be able to place current policy in a broader political and economic context and to find ways of getting the best from commissioning-led approaches – without necessarily believing that commissioning will be a panacea. We hope that this introductory textbook is a helpful starting point as part of this wider journey.

Further reading

At present, the strategic commissioning agenda is so new and emerging that there is no single set text on the topic. However, helpful overviews are provided by the following:

- Bamford, T. (2001) *Commissioning and purchasing*, London: Routledge (now a little dated, but a helpful and practical introduction).
- Figueras, J., Robinson, R. and Jakubowski, E. (2005) *Purchasing to improve health systems performance*, Maidenhead: Open University Press (an overview of international evidence from healthcare).
- Greve, C. (2008) *Contracting for public services*, London: Routledge (probably the most useful introduction, this book summarises some of the international experience/literature).
- Le Grand, J. (2003) *Motivation, agency and public policy: of knights and knaves, pawns and queens*, Oxford: Oxford University Press (this and the next book by Le Grand set out key arguments for and approaches to public sector reform).
- Le Grand, J. (2007) *The other invisible hand: delivering public services through choice and competition*, Princeton, NJ: Princeton University Press.
- McLaughlin, K., Osborne, S. and Ferlie, E. (eds) (2002) *New Public Management: current trends and future prospects*, London: Routledge (a more general book on NPM reforms).
- Macmillan, R. (2010) *The third sector delivering public services: an evidence review*, Birmingham: Third Sector Research Centre (a detailed but accessible review of the evidence surrounding third sector involvement in public service delivery, commissioning and procurement).
- Williams, I., Robinson, S. and Dickinson, H. (2011) *Rationing in health care: the theory and practice of priority setting*, Bristol: The Policy Press.

Useful websites

- Department of Health commissioning website (now archived): http://webarchive. nationalarchives.gov.uk/+/www.dh.gov.uk/en/Managingyourorganisation/ Commissioning/index.htm
- Institute of Commissioning Professionals: www.iocp.co.uk
- new economics foundation: www.neweconomics.org/projects/commissioning-public-benefit
- NHS Evidence: www.library.nhs.uk/commissioning/

Reflective exercises

1. Consider recent policy in the organisation/area where you work. To what extent does national policy promote a commissioning-led approach and how does this differ from previous policy? What difference has it made in practice to your role? What impact has it had for people using services?
2. How helpful is the concept of 'commissioning' as the 'conscience', 'brain' and 'eyes and ears' of the system and how do the insights that this provides differ from official definitions?
3. If you were starting with a blank sheet of paper, would you use 'commissioning' as a key tool if you were trying to design the perfect welfare system?
4. Given that public services are not starting with a blank sheet of paper, what advice would you give a new Secretary of State around the strengths/limitations of current commissioning and future reform?

References

Ashton, T., Cumming, J. and McLean, J. (2004) 'Contracting for health services in a public health system: the New Zealand experience', *Health Policy*, vol 69, pp 21-31.

Audit Commission (2007) *Healthy competition*, London: Audit Commission.

DH (Department of Health) (2007) *World class commissioning: vision*, London: DH.

DH (2010a) *Equity and excellence: liberating the NHS*, London: TSO.

DH (2010b) *Commissioning*, available online via www.dh.gov.uk/en/Managingyourorganisation/Commissioning/index.htm

Figueras, J., Robinson, R. and Jakubowski, E. (eds) (2005) *Purchasing to improve health systems performance*, Maidenhead: Open University Press.

Greve, C. (2008) *Contracting for public services*, London: Routledge.

Halvorson, G. (2007) *Health care reform now*, San Francisco, CA: Jossey-Bass.

Ham, C. (2008) *Health care commissioning in the international context: lessons from experience and evidence*, Birmingham: Health Services Management Centre.

Knapp, M., Hardy, B. and Forder, J. (2001) 'Commissioning for quality: ten years of social care markets in England', *Journal of Social Policy*, vol 30, no 2, pp 283-306.

Le Grand, J. (2003) *Motivation, agency and public policy*, Oxford: Oxford University Press.

Le Grand, J. (2007) *The other invisible hand: delivering public services through choice and competition*, Princeton, NJ: Princeton University Press.

Light, D. (1998) *Effective commissioning*, London: Office of Health Economics.

Mays, N. and Hand, K. (2000) *A review of options for health and disability support purchasing in New Zealand*, Working Paper, Wellington, New Zealand: New Zealand Treasury.

Mays, N., Wyke, S. and Evans, D. (eds) (2001) *The purchasing of health care by primary care organisations*, Buckingham: Open University Press.

McLaughlin, K., Osborne, S. and Ferlie, E. (eds) (2002) *New Public Management: current trends and future prospects*, London: Routledge.

Silow-Caroll, S. and Alteras, T. (2007) *Value-driven health care purchasing: four states that are ahead of the curve*, New York, NY: Commonwealth Fund.

Smith, J. and Mays, N. (2005) 'Primary care trusts: do they have a future?', *British Medical Journal*, vol 331, pp 1156-7.

Smith, J., Mays, N., Dixon, J., Goodwin, N., Lewis, R., McClelland, S., McLeod, H. and Wyke, S. (2004) *A review of the effectiveness of primary care-led commissioning in the UK NHS*, London: The Health Foundation.

Wade, E., Smith, J., Peck, E. and Freeman, T. (2006) *Commissioning in the reformed NHS: policy into practice*, Birmingham: Health Services Management Centre.

Williams, I., Robinson, S. and Dickinson, H. (2011) *Rationing in health care: the theory and practice of priority setting*, Bristol: The Policy Press.

Woodin, J. (2006) 'Health care commissioning and contracting', in K. Walshe and J. Smith (eds) *Healthcare management*, Maidenhead: Open University Press.

Part One

The commissioning cycle

ONE

New models of strategic commissioning

Tony Bovaird, Helen Dickinson and Kerry Allen

Summary

This chapter explores:
- the development of strategic commissioning across a range of public services;
- the limitations of strategic commissioning;
- key drivers for change;
- key implications and lessons learned.

The UK's New Labour government (1997-2010) continually wrestled to find ways of giving more emphasis to a mixed economy of public service provision, entailing greater externalisation. This underlying drive was often resisted, particularly at local level, but consistently re-emerged in government policy (Bovaird and Downe, 2006). This chapter chronicles the form that this drive took in the period from 2004 to 2010, which we characterise as a move to *'strategic commissioning'*. Whereas innovative approaches do not normally sweep through the public sector very rapidly, the move to strategic commissioning in the United Kingdom (UK) has been embraced by (almost) all central government ministries. Further, it is multi-sectoral – in the sense not only that it covers provision of welfare services by the public, private and third sectors, but also that it is also being applied to almost all subsectors of public services.

This chapter explores the development of strategic commissioning in a range of public services, its limitations and some of the drivers that have led this particular wave of innovation to spread much more quickly through the UK public sector than have most other innovations (particularly those that have been imposed by central government). It shows how a range of models (often developed in Whitehall) are being interpreted and redefined at the local level so that there is wide variation in the approaches to strategic commissioning actually being used in practice. The chapter ends by drawing some of the lessons emerging to date from experience with the UK strategic commissioning approach and exploring the implications for the era of fiscal restraint under the coalition government (in which service decommissioning is becoming the dominant trend). We start, however, by setting out an overview of the policy context. In doing so, we build on the brief introduction to this book by describing the move to commissioning of public services in the UK as occurring in two waves – the first in the late 1980s and early 1990s, and the second more recently, essentially since 2004. The main aim of the chapter is to place the more detailed debates that take place later in the book in a broader context, and so there is a series of links and cross-references to later chapters (which pick up specific issues in greater depth).

The move to commissioning ...

The original move to commissioning of public services came as part of the compulsory competitive tendering (CCT) approach in UK government from 1980, but this was further accentuated after the extension of CCT to a wide range of local government services after 1988 and to health services after 1991. This resulted in a mandatory split between public service planners and service purchasers, on the one hand, and the providers on the other – labelled the 'client–contractor split' in local government and the 'purchaser–provider split' in the National Health Service (NHS). This split was a key feature of the move to 'internal markets', which was a primary characteristic of the way that the New Public Management (NPM) played out in the UK at that time (see Ferlie et al, 1996).

While the government did evaluate the effects of CCT in local government during the early 1990s and published rather uncomfortable findings (Walsh, 1991; Walsh and Davis, 1993), it did not commission nor did it encourage the evaluation of the NHS reforms at that time (Dixon, 1998). The eventual evaluations that followed were summarised by Le Grand et al (1998, p 133):

> Most analysts of the internal market would agree ... the split between purchaser and provider, together with the development of contracts or service agreements between purchasers and providers that the market necessitated, were desirable innovations which should be retained in any future development of the system – despite the fact that, for some commentators, the extent of regulation excessively weakened the incentives inherent in the system.

They contrasted this (near) consensus with the disagreement over the desirability of the competition element of the internal markets policy. In Table 1.1 we summarise the pros and cons that were suggested in relation to the purchaser–provider split, drawing on the comments made widely not only in the practitioner literature but also in academic studies.

In the late 1990s, with the advent of New Labour, CCT was replaced by best value in local government and the principle of the internal market was partially rolled back in the NHS (only to be reinstated more fervently at a later date). Thus, the purchaser–provider split has continued to be an integral part of UK public sector reform.

Table 1.1: Pros and cons of the 'purchaser–provider split'

Advantages	Disadvantages
Promotes services that are systematically planned and based on assessed need	Reduces the role of providers in service development
Promotes output/outcome-orientation rather than activity-orientation	Promotes contract orientation – and therefore de facto input and process orientation (and, in any case, outcome orientation is often not practical)
Clarifies commissioner and provider roles and enables specialisation	May make strategic decisions more difficult because of insufficient commissioner knowledge of services in operation
Increases awareness of and pressure to reduce costs	Collaboration may be a more effective motivator than market-based competition – it may also be less costly than contracting, because of the transaction costs of formal tendering, contracting and monitoring regimes
Increases contestability which in turn reduces inefficiency (through cost or quality pressures)	Hindered by underdeveloped external markets
Increases scope for user voice *and* exit	Fractures responsibility for clients
Allows managers of provider units greater autonomy and freedom from 'micro-management' by commissioning managers	Exacerbates problems of coordination between agencies whose activities need to be highly interdependent
Symbolises change within an organisation and asserts a change in organisational culture	There may be a purely 'ceremonial' adoption of the purchaser–provider model by agencies, motivated perhaps by a desire to follow current fashion or to comply with the perceived expectations of dominant external stakeholders

... and then to strategic commissioning

The second wave of UK commissioning – the move to strategic commissioning – started in earnest with the *Every child matters* White Paper in 2003 (HM Treasury, 2003), leading to the Children Act 2004 and the development of an associated strategic commissioning framework over 2005-06. This example was quickly followed by other government departments, particularly those working in personal services (such as health, social care, local government services, the criminal justice system and services for the workless). While some government departments largely remained aloof (for example, the Department for International Development and, until recently, the Department for Environment, Food and Rural Affairs [DEFRA]), strategic commissioning became the 'main show in town' for many areas of public service (see Table 1.2). Indeed, as Walters (2009) has commented, the language around 'commissioning' has come to dominate political discourse. He points out that references to 'commissioning' in *Hansard* (the daily report of debates and committee meetings in Parliament) jumped from 12 mentions in 1988, to 248 mentions in 1997, to 1,000 mentions in 2007. However, it should be noted that strategic commissioning has not been embraced with the same enthusiasm across all areas of the UK. In the field of health, the

—

Table 1.2: The evolution of strategic commissioning in the UK public sector since 2003

Date	Title	Policy area	Source	Role of commissioning
2003-06	*Every child matters* White Paper (HM Treasury, 2003), Children Act 2004 and *Joint planning and commissioning framework for children, young people and maternity services* (HM Government, 2006)	Children's and young people's services	Cross-government (Department of Health [DH], Department for Children, Schools and Families [DCSF] and Department for Communities and Local Government [DCLG])	Essentially procurement (of five statutory outcomes)
2006	*Health reform in England: update and commissioning framework* (DH, 2006a)	Primary healthcare	DH	Whole planning and management cycle (except perhaps delivery)
2006-08	*Strong and prosperous communities* White Paper (DCLG, 2006), followed by guidance on strategic commissioning (DCLG, 2008)	All local public services	DCLG	Whole planning and management cycle (except delivery)
2006	*Partnership in public services* (OTS, 2006)	Public services involving third sector organisations	Office of the Third Sector (OTS)	Whole planning and management cycle (except delivery)
2007	*Commissioning framework for health and well-being* (DH, 2007a)	Contribution of all public services to health and well-being outcomes and health inequalities	DH and DCLG	Whole planning and management cycle (except delivery)
2007	*World class commissioning* (DH, 2007b)	Health	DH	Whole planning and management cycle (except delivery)
2008	*The DWP's commissioning strategy* (Cave, n.d.)	Services for workless people	Department for Work and Pensions (DWP)	Planning of programmes for delivery by 'prime contractors'
2009	*Achieving better outcomes: commissioning in children's services* (Commissioning Support Programme, 2009)	Children's and young people's services	Cross-government (DH, DCSF and DCLG)	'Place shaping for local outcomes' – including whole planning and management cycle (except delivery)

Welsh and Scottish governments have actively sought to distance their systems from commissioning and a purchaser–provider split and towards planner/purchaser structures (Dickinson and Ham, 2008).

In early 2010, we undertook a survey of the current 'state of the art' in strategic commissioning in UK government (Bovaird et al, 2010). We found that most government departments that dealt with local public services had developed an overall approach to and framework for 'strategic commissioning'; although some departments, such as DEFRA, admitted that they had only just started to take this approach. However, in practice there was a significant divergence in the approaches actually used and the differences between them had not been fully identified and resolved in the evolving debate before the new coalition government took office in May 2010.

Strategic commissioning: what does it actually mean?

Models of commissioning

No standard definition of 'strategic commissioning' has yet emerged. In the strategic commissioning cycle outlined in *Every child matters* (HM Treasury, 2003), 'commissioning' refers explicitly to services (often with pooled resources) from providers, and lies within the cycle between planning the pattern of desired services and planning for workforce and market development (see Figure 1.1). However,

Figure 1.1: The *Every child matters* commissioning cycle

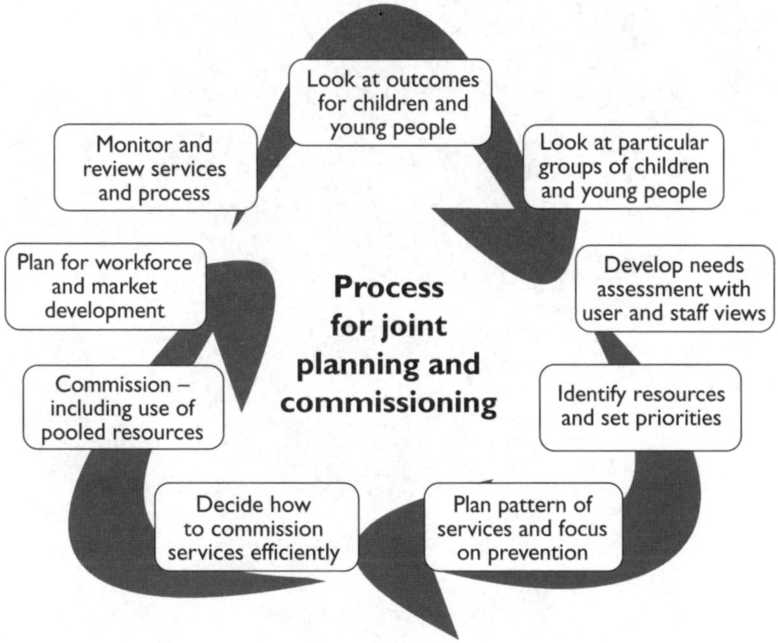

Source: HM Treasury (2003)

the Cabinet Office (2006, p 4) defines commissioning much more widely as 'the cycle of assessing the needs of people in an area, designing and then securing appropriate service'. A similar approach was taken by the Department of Health (DH, 2007a, p 94), which defined commissioning as 'the full set of activities that local authorities and Primary Care Trusts (PCTs) undertake to make sure that services meet the health and social care needs of individuals and communities' (see Figure 1.2). Neither of these definitions explicitly separates the service commissioning role from the service delivery role, although in both cases it is clear that such a separation was intended to be assumed. Both definitions mark a significant extension in the functions included, compared to the definition used just a little earlier in *Every child matters*.

Figure 1.2:The commissioning cycle in world class commissioning (DH)

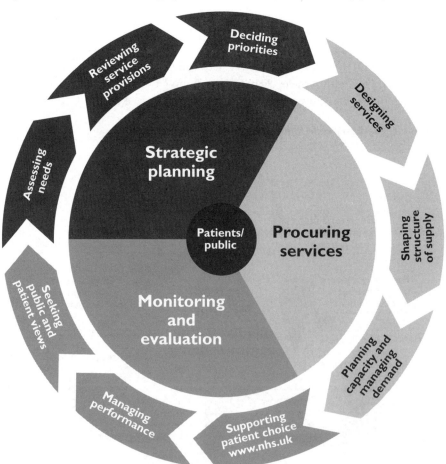

Source: http://www.ic.nhs.uk/commissioning

Commissioning increasingly began to be seen as the primary means of driving improvement in the NHS as the impact of the target regime began to wane (Allen et al, 2009). By 2008, the DH approach of 'world class commissioning' in England (see Figure 1.2) clearly distinguished the core underlying functions of 'planning', 'procurement' and 'monitoring and evaluation' and made it clear that commissioning was entirely separate from delivery – essentially, 'commissioning' was every part of the rational management cycle *other than* delivery. However, the Secretary of State for Health caused a furore in September 2009 when he announced in a speech that the NHS was the 'provider of choice' (Vize, 2009), although this was later clarified as referring specifically to services currently provided by the NHS – where PCTs wish to commission new services, or new service models, or to increase patient choice, this should be subject to open competition.

The approach to strategic commissioning continues to differ further between service sectors. In its 2006 White Paper entitled *Strong and prosperous communities*, the Department for Communities and Local Government (DCLG, 2006) set out a wide-ranging role for strategic commissioning of local government services, locating it as a vital part of 'place shaping'. Place shaping is defined as building a vision of how to respond to and address a locality's problems and challenges in a coordinated way, including issues such as economic futures, demographic shifts, climate change, offending, and cohesive communities. Again, it insisted on the separation of commissioning and provision, 'thus enabling the LA [local authority] and the LSP [local strategic partnership] to be the champion of the citizen and service improvement' (DCLG, 2006, paras 5.67-5.68). It stressed the need for local authorities to work more through partnerships in their strategic commissioning – 'rather than delivering services directly themselves' (DCLG, 2006, para 5.6). Various reasons were given for this, including:

- better use of competition and alternative providers as a driver for innovation;
- a more holistic approach to commissioning services – not a simplistic approach to outsourcing;
- optimal solutions that balance quality and value for money;
- the key role of procurement in providing high-quality services and extending choice;
- encouraging more providers in the market.

However, confusingly, in its discussion of the elements of the commissioning cycle, it included delivery, as well as identifying needs, planning, sourcing and performance management.

The final commissioning cycle illustrated here is from the DWP (Figure 1.3). This has become increasingly powerful in Whitehall, because it embodies a strong commitment to the use of 'prime contractors' who essentially undertake most of the supply chain management (which in other models is done by the commissioning bodies). As can be seen from Figure 1.3, the cycle puts considerable

Figure 1.3: The Department of Work and Pensions commissioning cycle

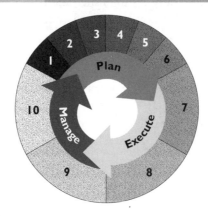

The Commissioning Cycle is at the heart of our strategy

1. **Demand analysis**
   Analysis of the likely demand for contracted provision in terms of the numbers of people likely to use the services.

2. **Market capacity**
   Is there enough capacity in the market to deliver the services we require?

3. **Resource analysis**
   Does the Department have the resources in terms of budget, people and skills to procure the services it needs effectively?

4. **Risk analysis**
   Highlight risks to commissioning a delivery of contracted services. For example, risks might include increased demand of services and capital constrained providers unable to grow to meet demand.

5. **Strategic plan/Commissioning pipeline**
   Bringing together all the available information into a single strategic commission plan outlining how DWP will deliver its objectives through the commissioning of services.

6. **Contract design**
   Designing contracts that incentivise providers to deliver what we want. i.e. deliver sustained job outcomes and not to 'cream' or 'park' customers.

7. **Contract implementation**
   Put strategy into action through commissioning.

8. **Provider development**
   Support provider development and promote best practice, for example through the Provider Forum. This might include helping providers wanting to expand or leave the market.

9. **Contract management**
   Metrics should capture how well DWP issues and manages its contracts. This may include stakeholder satisfaction, quality of our data etc.

10. **Performance management**
    Monitor provider performance in terms of outcomes against targets and each other; as well as customer feedback and reports on provider capability (Ofsted).

Source: Cave, n.d.

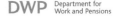
DWP Department for
Work and Pensions

emphasis on market management issues, such as analysing market capacity, risk analysis of providers, provider development and contract management. However, Figure 1.3 also illustrates how easy it is for the language around 'commissioning' to become confusing: step 7 – 'contract implementation' – talks of 'putting strategy into action through commissioning', when this would more usually be described as part of the 'procurement' function (we reflect further on the distinctions between functions within commissioning models below).

Intentions for user-centric and outcomes-oriented processes

A key claim in the New Labour government's approach to strategic commissioning was that it involves the 'public in the design of services, especially those who might otherwise be marginalized' (DCLG, 2006, para 2.21; see also Chapter Nine, this volume). For example, the DCLG (2006, para 2.21) stresses the need for local authorities and suppliers to work together to provide contractual incentives for both external and in-house providers to meet expectations of users. Similar user-centric policies are stressed in the government's approach to strategic commissioning in health. The DH (2007, p 10) *Commissioning framework for health and well-being* promised '[a] shift towards services that are personal, sensitive to individual needs' and that 'people' (patients and the public) would be at the centre of the commissioning cycle.

The government has also presented strategic commissioning as being outcome driven (see Chapter Seven, this volume). For example, HM Government (2006) states that the *Joint planning and commissioning framework for children, young people and maternity services* will be focused on achieving the five outcomes from *Every child matters* (consisting of 'being healthy', 'staying safe', 'enjoying and achieving', 'making a positive contribution' and 'economic well-being'). It stresses the need to join up services so that they produce better outcomes, partly by ensuring that contracts are based increasingly on outcomes. The DCLG guidance on *Creating strong, safe and prosperous communities* (DCLG, 2008) explicitly states that commissioning involves (among other functions) strategically planning for services that deliver sustainable outcomes, securing services and outcomes and monitoring the delivery of outcomes. *Our health, our care, our say* (DH, 2006b) built on the social care Green Paper of the previous year (DH, 2005) to set out the outcomes that health and social care services should be working towards for adults in England. Furthermore, the government has proposed these principles not simply for its own services, suggesting the need for their extension to the third sector's role in the delivery of public services. The former Office of the Third Sector (OTS, 2006) proposed a set of 'commissioning principles' for government in its dealing with the third sector, which included putting outcomes for users at the heart of the strategic planning process. The important theme here is that the focus of strategic commissioning should be away from measuring outputs or activities and towards the actual difference that these activities make. Further, these outcome measures should be defined by individuals themselves, rather than the statutory body.

Dissemination of the strategic commissioning approach to local public services

Whereas many previous innovations at central government level have tended to have had only limited take-up, particularly at local level (Martin et al, 2009), the move to strategic commissioning has been widespread and largely unopposed, at least in the public debate in England (it has been more challenged in devolved UK governments particularly in the field of health). In this section we examine what has led this particular wave of innovation to spread much more quickly through the UK public sector than most other innovations (particularly those that are government led), before moving on to look at some of the ways in which strategic commissioning has been delivered at a local level. We argue that the lack of clarity at a national level has led to strategic commissioning being implemented in a range of different ways.

At the central government level, drivers of the strategic commissioning approach included the Gershon efficiency savings programme from 2004 onwards and the fiscal crisis from 2008 onwards. However, this does not provide a full explanation for the acceptance of strategic commissioning. It does not explain, for example, why departments such as DEFRA were so slow to turn to strategic commissioning in their environmental improvement programmes – something that only began to happen systematically from 2009 onwards. Similarly, the commitment to a mixed economy of provision, a constant theme of New Labour since 1997 (Bovaird and Downe, 2006), with its concomitant pressures to separate purchasers and providers, was clearly not the determining factor in the DH in 2009, when the Secretary of State overturned much of the logic of this position by declaring that NHS delivery units continued to be 'the providers of choice' for NHS commissioners. The very variety of approaches adopted in Whitehall, as set out in Table 1.2, suggests that there were no universal drivers (and certainly no single organising logic) behind the move to strategic commissioning in central government.

At the local level, some of the take-up of the strategic commissioning approach has been because of its embedding in legal requirements – for example the arrangements for Children's Trusts and for world class commissioning. However, this does not extend to other local public services. Indeed, the Audit Commission approach to Comprehensive Area Assessment in local public services and to the Use of Resources judgements in local government and the NHS does not make specific mention of strategic commissioning, so that local public agencies have considerable freedom in how they choose to arrange for strategic commissioning (Audit Commission et al, 2010). This freedom has resulted in substantial levels of innovation in how strategic commissioning plays out at the local level. In a research study for a joint Local Government Association and Confederation of British Industry inquiry into strategic commissioning (LGA and CBI, 2009), subsequently updated in a study for the National Audit Office (Bovaird et al, 2010), we found a range of approaches at the local level, and a range of views about the advantages and disadvantages of these approaches (see Table 1.3).

In addition to those set out already in this section, there are a number of national commissioning models that do not vary across local areas. For example, in England there is a national-level commissioning infrastructure in place for highly specialised healthcare services such as organ transplants, children's heart and neurosurgery, specialised burn care, some types of stem cell therapy, rare neuromuscular disease and cancer of the retina. Services are commissioned by the

Table 1.3: Different types of commissioning, advantages and disadvantages

Type of commissioning	Explanation and examples	Advantages	Disadvantages
Single agency commissioning	Where a single organisation is responsible for all stages of commissioning services. Public sector organisation commissioning, procuring and contracting a service entirely by itself eg for leisure centres, street cleaning, prisons etc, primary care organisation/PCT commissioning (Smith et al, 2004), single practice-based commissioning in health (Smith et al, 2005)	– Simple to coordinate – May be able to react more quickly to changing circumstances – May be less complex for service users, who can see clearly which agency is responsible for commissioning	– Ignores interdependencies between different agencies with commissioning responsibilities for similar outcomes – Less opportunity for knowledge transfer between commissioning agencies – Less able to offer sizeable contracts that yield economies of scale
'Service integrator' commissioning	Where the commissioner(s) appoint a prime contractor as broker for the subcontractor network (the 'service integrator' model) (eg DWP commissioning New Deal through private sector prime contractors). These services differ between funding schemes and between areas, depending on which prime contractor has won the contract for a particular programme in that area	– Simple, for the strategic commissioner – Reduces risk of commissioner mismanaging the supply chain – May help to bring the skills of the third sector, through more flexibly managed subcontractor networks	– Increases risk from choosing 'wrong' prime contractor – May exclude small, specialist, existing providers – May squeeze out good local providers who are not in the prime contractor's network – Reduces customer choice and control

(continued)

Table 1.3: (continued)

Type of commissioning	Explanation and examples	Advantages	Disadvantages
Area-based joint commissioning	Where several organisations form a partnership, alliance or other collaboration, taking joint responsibility for the commissioning of services. There are many variations of this model. Examples include: LSP-led strategic commissioning/ commissioning for place (DCLG, 2009a); joint or integrated commissioning (Smith et al, 2004); multi-practice or locality health commissioning (Smith et al, 2004); lead commissioning (Smith et al, 2004); neighbourhood-led commissioning (Bovaird, 2009); radical community commissioning, with participatory budgeting (eg through 'community chests', or through young people's services commissioning panels with user representation) (Bovaird, 2009); inter-area (sub-regional) commissioning (eg at city region level or through Multi-Area Agreements) etc	– Joint commissioning reduces overlap and duplications, creating scope for efficiency savings – Identifies areas of insufficient coordination of standards and targets – Enables economies of scale – Helps third sector to identify more effective roles for its potential contribution through a clear statement of future requirements in the area – Gives an area-based focus to outcomes – (For inter-area commissioning) enables a joined-up approach to issues crossing area and agency boundaries and allows faster dissemination of best practice	– Action relies entirely on partnership working on a voluntary basis because responsibility for any spending remains with separate agencies potentially raising issues of accountability – Different performance management regimes mean that different parts of government (and hence local agencies) prioritise different outcomes and budgets (these require local initiative and central action) – Bringing together different organisational cultures takes management time and effort – May result in such large scale contracts that third sector organisations and small firms are not able to bid realistically for them – (For inter-area commissioning) may override local priorities in order to achieve a sub-regional perspective on service requirements and governance and accountability may be more complicated across geographical boundaries

(continued)

Table 1.3: (continued)

Type of commissioning	Explanation and examples	Advantages	Disadvantages
User-led commissioning	There is increasing awareness among commissioners of the benefits of service user involvement in strategic commissioning. The move towards personalisation and the direct purchase of services by individuals or neighbourhoods demonstrate the most extreme variants of this approach. Examples of user-led commissioning include individual patient purchasing, patient choice and user-led commissioning (Smith et al, 2004; LGA and CBI, 2009); extension of individual budgets; vouchers for all or part of purchase (Bovaird, 2009); user and community co-production (of service commissioning and delivery) (Bovaird and Loeffler, 2009)	– Puts users, rather than professionals in control – Allows users to tailor the service for their own needs rather than having outcomes dictated by others – Gives users some choice of service deliverer – May allow users to 'top-up' the service to increase the volume or quality of service received – May allow the purchasing agency to negotiate favourable deals with potential providers (at a maximum under vouchers)	– Not all users value choice and some could regard involvement as a burden – It may not be possible to meet all users' expectations – Users who make choices that are not within the scheme criteria are either opening the scheme up to accusations of abuse or are stopped from making their preferred choices, which makes the choice element of the scheme seem illusory to them – As with all choice programmes, choices based on irrelevant or misinformed criteria may introduce a destabilising dynamic to the overall service system – Block purchase options that reduce costs could be threatened
Investment-driven commissioning	Models of investment-based commissioning aim to inject new capital and deliver improved outcomes. The strength of investment-driven commissioning is seen as early communication of expert knowledge between authorities and varied partners. Examples of investment-driven commissioning include: Building Schools for the Future (BSF) and Local Education Partnerships, Local Infrastructure Finance Trusts (LIFT), and Housing and Communities Total Capital Programme	– Bringing partners together to act as joint commissioners as well as service deliverers ensures a more holistic approach to service planning and design – This allows private sector partners to contribute project planning and design expertise at an earlier stage. – The LIFT and BSF programmes were also supported by a national programme management organisation, and by central co-ordinating bodies, Partnerships for Health and Partnerships for Schools, which assisted with procurement/knowledge transfer across projects	– Potential inflexibility built into initial partnership arrangements (although likely to be more flexible than similar PFI schemes) – Expensive capital, cost of setting up agreements

National Commissioning Group (NCG), which oversees and supports 10 regional specialised commissioning groups. The NCG also advises government on NHS services that are best commissioned nationally, rather than locally.

Taken together with Table 1.2, it is clear that the general consensus in Whitehall around the need for strategic commissioning has not played out as a single, homogenous approach, at either the central or the local level. This can be seen especially clearly in the case of the DH, which during the period after 2007 was associated with a series of strategic commissioning models, each of them significantly different and with little attempt to integrate them into a single approach:

- *world class commissioning* for the NHS, which was a centrally driven model with relatively little local variation;
- *commissioning for children's services*, jointly with the DCSF and the DCLG, which allowed significant local variation;
- *personalisation and individual budgets for adult social care*, which greatly reduced the role of public sector strategic commissioners in shaping services, in order to increase the decision-making role of service users.

It seems likely, therefore, that the high level of innovation in finding new models of strategic commissioning derives at least partly from differences of approach across government departments. These differences have left more room for innovation at the local level by local government and other local service deliverers than would have been possible under an entirely 'joined-up' central government agenda. Some areas of commissioning have more latitude than others. For example, although PCTs have previously been constrained under world class commissioning in the NHS, even here, some local PCTs have taken seriously the government's stated commitment to Local Area Agreements (LAAs), so that they have put more emphasis on the LAA targets they have agreed through joint strategic commissioning at the local level than on their achievement of centrally determined 'vital signs' in the DH performance management framework. Moreover, some of these local innovations have stimulated significant interest at central government level (for example, user and community co-production, participatory budgeting and neighbourhood-led commissioning), leading to national pilot schemes.

Problems and limitations of strategic commissioning

As with any managerial practice, there are clearly limitations and drawbacks to the spread of strategic commissioning. In this section, we look at some of the problems that still exist or are emerging in the current UK approaches to strategic commissioning. While many of the potential issues identified from the purchaser–provider split in Table 1.1 continue to be problematic, the debate around commissioning in 2010 focused on a rather different set of concerns.

The debate over meaning

What is meant by 'commissioning' is not always clear and differs across government departments. Indeed, the Public Administration Select Committee (2008, para 38) of the House of Commons commented:

> If there is no common understanding of what commissioning means, that can only be a barrier to effective relationships. Government and the private and third sector need to come to a commonly accepted definition of commissioning if it is to continue to be the State's preferred method of interacting with the sector.

As demonstrated above, the rhetoric about separating the commissioner and provider roles has not always meant in practice that a clear separation has been achieved (or, indeed, desired). Many of the commissioning cycles in central government models have not made the split clear, while even when it has been said to be important in the models, it has been contradicted in policy or practice – as in the case of the Secretary of State for Health in 2009. As a result, there are still many in government who confuse the distinction between commissioning, purchasing, procurement and contracting.

The commissioning–purchasing split is most clearly visible where there are individual budgets, so that the commissioner is clearly the individual and the purchaser is the public agency making this budget available to the individuals concerned (see Chapter Eleven, this volume). A similar distinction is clear where 'community chests' are made available to neighbourhoods, communities or stakeholder groups for funding of projects (often match-funded), which they themselves can partly determine. However, the distinction is not always so clear cut; where partnerships commission jointly, using a variety of funding sources (for example, pooled budgets, grants from the European Union or Whitehall, individual agency budgets), the separate roles (and accountabilities) of the commissioners and purchasers can be hard to disentangle (see Chapter Ten, this volume).

As we have seen above, the commissioning–procurement distinction is one that has been particularly difficult for government to make – and remains so. Indeed, there is a widespread view that 'commissioning' essentially means procuring external contractors. Reinforcing this concern, Adam Sharples, a senior British civil servant has recently written: 'Traditionally, government bodies deliver services to citizens, but with commissioning, the public body contracts with an outside organization to deliver those services' (Bourgon, 2011, p 25). What is particularly damaging about such confusion is that the belief that 'commissioning' is the same as externalisation has soured the general attitude towards commissioning of many stakeholders, particularly trades unions and politicians. Again, in Wales in early 2008, Health Boards were instructed by the Welsh Assembly Government (2008, p 1) not to use the phrase 'commissioning' (using 'planning' instead) because the

---

commissioning approach had turned out to be 'provider driven', and 'in reality no real market exists for the majority of care'.

Often it is not simply that these concepts are not conceptually distinguished from one another – even where they are, procurement and contracting processes are not aligned. There are a number of major problems for commissioning arising from current developments in procurement. In particular, the imperative to improve value for money in the current fiscal crisis is leading to pressures for letting bigger, longer contracts to smaller numbers of providers, in order both to reduce the transaction costs of procurement and to ensure that bidders are able to offer better value for money through economies of scale and scope. There are major concerns that this may lead to squeezing out high-quality but small local providers, whether in the private or third sector. There is also a concern – although this is likely to be longer term – that it may result eventually in overdependence on a few major independent providers, who may behave in a quasi-monopolistic fashion towards the commissioners and who would be able to impose highly unfavourable terms on subcontractors, decreasing the long-term diversity of quality providers (Horne and Baeck, 2010). While regulation may help to alleviate some of these problems (for example through the MERLIN standard for good supply chain management, which the DWP imposes on its prime contractors), there is some scepticism as to how well the public sector can actually intervene lower down the supply chain. Similarly, any move to longer-term contracts in order to tempt contractors to offer larger short-term savings might eventually result in damaging inflexibility in services.

More fundamentally, the imperative to achieve large short-term savings in the commissioning process might well result in design and letting of savings-oriented rather than value-for-money-oriented contracts, might slow down the gradual movement in procurement towards 'dialogue' and relational contracts (rather than specification-based contracts), might reinforce the attempt to focus on squeezing more costs out of service specifications (rather than fundamentally challenging current service perspectives, which are fixed on problem alleviation rather than problem prevention) and might drive short-term 'provider-led' solutions rather than co-production through 'user-led' (for example expert patients) or 'community-led' (for example community management of public assets) approaches, which may take longer and require some pump-priming funding.

Balancing competing policy agendas

The move to personalisation has reinforced the move to outcome-based commissioning, since service users can be expected to understand their own desired outcomes better than can be encapsulated in any user needs assessment (see Chapter Eleven, this volume, for an alternative view to the discussion here). It also contributes to the move towards user choice and a more competitive market for providers. However, it also has limitations. It is most justified where the key problem addressed in the commissioning process is the income (or wealth)

—

deficiency of service users. In such cases, individual budgets are simply a way of making the over-crude welfare benefits system sensitive to personal circumstances.

However, some services are provided publicly not simply because their recipients cannot afford to buy them in the marketplace – where there are market failures (for example where there is low competition in provision, where there is *no* market provision, or where the choices of users would have unfortunate knock-on effects on other citizens), then public provision may be justified and individual budgets would not be an adequate replacement. Here we can see the working of the vicious circle of provision failure; because arrangements in civil society cannot meet all the needs of some citizens, they have to seek to buy services external to the family and their networks (that is, from the marketplace). Because all markets have some failures, and some citizens in need have insufficient income and wealth to be able to buy adequate provision from the market, some of these needs are better met by state intervention (which may include redistribution and regulation rather than direct provision). Because all government intervention gives rise to some failure, there is a need for citizens to make use of civil society or the market to remedy the deficiencies in government intervention. And so on. In other words, the role of personalisation and individual budgets is to help provide the right balance between civil society, the market economy and the public sector in meeting user and social needs. Proponents of personalisation and individual budgets have sometimes missed this point and given pre-eminence to this approach to commissioning, which airbrushes out our long experience with the deficiencies of user-led demand and market-based provision.

Needs assessment and performance management

The move to joint needs assessment within collaborative models of strategic commissioning has been widely welcomed as a way of gauging holistic needs of actual and potential service users (see Chapter Two, this volume). However, it has also given rise to concerns about the inward-looking nature of this process, giving as it does a monopoly to state agencies in deciding what 'needs' are. Horne and Baeck (2010) suggest that there is a need both to bring in more potential agencies that can undertake these needs assessments, including user-led third sector organisations, and to ensure that needs assessments (for areas, for services as a whole and for specific individuals) are more open to challenge from service users and their communities, even to the point of sometimes leading the commissioning process and managing the day-to-day delivery of local services, as a DCLG (2009b) internal consultation paper suggested. More generally, there is now increasing debate about the insufficiency of a 'needs assessment' that is simply gauging 'needs for service' – a more holistic approach would also gauge an individual's ability and willingness to contribute to the community. This would mean shifting from a 'deficit' model of what is wrong with individuals and communities, to strengthening their aspirations and removing the obstacles they face in achieving their desired outcomes – moving the focus from structure and process and spending on services, towards investing in people and community outcomes. Such a 'resources and assets' assessment would allow citizens' expertise, knowledge, skills and willingness to give time to helping others, so forming a building block in a more systematic approach to co-production within the 'Big Society', and thus helping to fulfill the needs that individuals have to make a positive contribution in their lives (one of the national outcomes that both the DH and the DWP have specified for adult social services). It would parallel the move to giving more control and influence over resources to local communities, through personal and participatory budgeting, questioning not only current local public services but also the role of local authorities, their partners and their suppliers, and their relationship with the communities they serve, in a 'place-based budgeting' perspective.

The commissioning models considered in this chapter have almost all been related to existing performance management regimes – for example, the 'vital signs' performance reporting system for PCTs and the LAA performance management regime for LSPs (including local authorities, PCTs, police and fire authorities). This means that the commissioning frameworks are integrated into existing systems of accountability and therefore do not impose a separate burden on the agencies involved. There are, however, several ways in which current performance management systems bring about dysfunctional effects in the practical working of commissioning approaches. First, there is sometimes a rather poor fit between the commissioning model and the performance management framework associated with it. This is especially the case where commissioning models emphasise outcome-based approaches, which are not fully reflected in the performance management regimes. A glaring example of this occurs in children's services, where no indicators in the national indicator set pick up one of the five statutory outcomes ('enjoy'). Since the performance management regime is often more visible and drives operational decisions, this may mean that strategic commissioning appears rather theoretical or even partially irrelevant to managers (although its rhetorical value in achieving 'buy-in' from stakeholders may remain important).

A second danger occurs where there are conflicting performance management regimes within any given commissioning model – most evident where commissioning models bridge across government departments. For example, the commissioning model for the *Joint planning and commissioning framework for children, young people and maternity services* (HM Government, 2006) covered the territory of both the former DCSF and the DH. The performance management regimes applied by these two departments were interpreted by many agencies at the local level as driving them in different directions, with unfortunate results for clarity of resource allocation and action. However, strategic commissioning might not be simply a mechanism to bring about a set of clear changes – on occasion it may be more a way of drawing a range of stakeholders together in relation to a specific agenda (Dickinson, 2010), so that ambiguous or difficult-to-measure outcomes are not a major issue. For both these reasons, it is not surprising that there is little evidence yet that strategic commissioning has brought about significant improvements in organisational performance (Bovaird et al, 2010).

Government reports have focused on the potential benefits of outcome-based commissioning and procurement (for example that it gives clear strategic direction to providers, while allowing freedom to innovate; that it promotes preventative approaches; and that it focuses on the need for service integration across and within providers). However, it is clear that outcome-based approaches have not yet become as fully embedded in UK public sector practice as they have in the rhetoric. The lack of integrated services and integrated use of public assets was painfully highlighted by the Total Place pilots in 2009-10 – and although these problems may now be tackled in the new place-based budgeting approaches of the coalition government, the obstacles clearly remain enormous. Perhaps most challenging of all is the design of a staged process by which the outcomes considered in commissioning can be given weight in procurement decision making, and then translated in some form to the incentive system for rewarding providers (for example through outcome-related payments or a clear system for assessing success against desired outcomes at contract review stage). While outcome-based contract payment is now slowly spreading from the worklessness agenda, where it was pioneered by the DWP, to offender management and some aspects of children's and mental health services, it seems likely that it will always be a contentious and risky way of incentivising providers of public services, given the large number of external variables that affect outcomes.

Implications for future public services management in the UK

As we have argued in this chapter, notions of strategic commissioning are inevitably closely linked with particular political administrations. Therefore a change of government potentially signals changes in strategic commissioning policy and models. The new coalition government was at first rather coy about its stance on strategic commissioning. Indeed, in one Whitehall department (DCLG) the phrase 'commissioning' was not used for some time after the election in May 2010, although in others it remained alive and well. Despite this, the idea of strategic commissioning does seem to have become embedded in the culture, structure and processes of public services in the UK during the past two decades. Indeed, a DCLG (2009b) internal consultation paper advocated extension of the commissioning approach to local 'place-based services' (for example, waste management, leisure, culture and libraries, regeneration, transport and regulatory services) in order that a common platform could be built for service improvement and transformation. NHS reform in particular has also continued to stress the importance of this way of working through the championing of general practitioner-led commissioning. Under whatever label 'commissioning' goes in the future, it seems likely that the kernel of most of the features reported in this chapter will remain – the commissioner–provider split (although it is still unclear whether this will be more or less 'hard' than in the last two decades), joint needs analysis, market testing, market development and management, performance management (although probably less target fixated than in the last decade) and significant user and citizen involvement in all or most phases of the commissioning cycle. While the relative prominence of these features of the commissioning approach has varied over time, the lesson of the past 20 years has been that they are never far away and tend to come back into fashion again on a regular basis.

A year before the General Election, some policy advisers in the Conservative Party started talking about 'results' and ostentatiously made little reference to 'outcomes'. However, there has appeared to be no let-up in the concern for achieving outcomes rather than simply outputs in the coalition government's pronouncements since it came to power. In any case, whatever they are called, the outcomes that have come to be identified and placed in the centre of strategic commissioning during the last decade are likely to remain important and to drive planning and action in public services in the near future. However, they may become more implicit than under the last administration – for example, the personalisation agenda will allow users to determine their desired outcomes for themselves. The measured outcomes of public services may be less often published for public debate. For example, the government has decided that the national indicator set will no longer be collected and published by Whitehall, although local public agencies are free to continue to collect and publish the data locally. This was ostensibly on grounds of allowing more localised priorities to determine which outcomes are measured, but with the obvious knock-on benefit that the effects of public expenditure cuts on outcomes will be less easy to track. Nevertheless, information about outcomes is still likely to be used in some form for prioritisation decisions at political level, both nationally and locally.

In the next phase of public expenditure planning and management in the UK, it is clear that strategic decommissioning of services will play a very prominent role (see Chapters Three and Five, this volume; see also Williams et al, 2011). As part of this, the government has emphasised that radical solutions will be entertained, and that, in particular, there will be a much greater emphasis on engaging third sector organisations and civil society in commissioning and decommissioning processes, as part of the 'Big Society'. Both the radical reconfiguration of remaining public services and the drawing in of contributions from citizens and communities in new ways will involve major innovation. On the positive side, this generates the possibility of major improvements in the achievement of outcomes that really matter and the junking of processes and outputs that do not matter to citizens. However, it also brings with it the reality of disruption and the risk of serious unintended consequences. To cope with these successfully, it will be necessary to see the changes during the next few years as a major series of untried experiments, with careful tracking mechanisms honed to detect quickly what is working and what is not working. While the performance management system in the UK has been developed to a stage where it is probably the most advanced in the world, there is a danger that the coalition government may partially dismantle it, just when it is most needed.

—

A major experimental programme of public service change, based on a rich set of new models of outcome-based commissioning, procurement and delivery is potentially a very exciting departure. However, the positive embracing of experiments, with the open and honest prior admission that many pathways will turn out to be blind alleys, has not been a hallmark of the UK government's approach to commissioning to date. Experiment, acceptance of 'potentially justifiable' risk and admission of 'revealing failure' have generally been perceived very negatively by most key stakeholders (particularly chief executives, corporate directors, politicians and leaders of the voluntary and community sector). This may therefore be the most challenging period so far in the development of the commissioning model for public services.

Conclusion

Strategic commissioning has emerged as an important component of policy across a number of policy domains of the UK. Although an interest in strategic commissioning has persisted across these different domains, a range of different models has emerged, which conceptualises this in different ways. We have argued that how strategic commissioning is treated is not consistent, although various features are common across these domains. Yet despite this sustained interest there is still little evidence that strategic commissioning has improved outcomes – it may be that the value of strategic commissioning is as much symbolic as practical or rational.

Acknowledgements

The research on which this chapter is based was undertaken as part of several projects funded by external bodies. The analysis of current government models of commissioning was undertaken as part of a review of commissioning across government (for the National Audit Office). The review of new models of strategic commissioning was begun in a project funded jointly by the Local Government Association and the Confederation of British Industry.

Further reading

This is a rapidly emerging area with few helpful overviews/background texts. However, helpful contributions include:

- Horne, M. and Baeck, P. (2010) *Shaking up commissioning*, London: Innovation Unit and NESTA.
- LGA and CBI (Local Government Association and Confederation of British Industry) (2009) *Commissioning strategically for better public services across local government*, London: CBI.

Useful websites

Strategic commissioning models can be found on the websites of the following governmental departments:

- Department for Education: www.education.gov.uk/
- Department of Health: www.dh.gov.uk/
- Department for Communities and Local Government: www.communities. gov.uk/

Reflective exercises

1. Give *your* definitions of 'strategic commissioning', 'procurement' and 'contracting'. For each term, find one example of a public agency that appears to use your definition (or a very similar definition) – and another public agency whose definition appears significantly different from your definition. Why do you think that these differences have occurred – for example, because of the user groups that they serve, the stakeholder groups involved in the process or for other reasons?
2. To what extent have the problems with the purchaser–provider split, as outlined in Table 1.1, been overcome in the strategic commissioning process with which you are most familiar? Have new problems from the purchaser–provider split arisen in relation to this strategic commissioning process? If so, how would you propose to overcome them?
3. For one service with which you are familiar (or for which you can get ready access to relevant material), set out the key outcomes that you believe are relevant to strategic commissioning. Demonstrate how you would build these outcomes into the commissioning, procurement and contracting processes. In the case of outcomes that are difficult to build into one or more of these processes, how would you treat them?
4. For one service with which you are familiar (or for which you can get ready access to relevant material), set out the performance management regime (or regimes) under which the different stakeholders are held accountable. To what extent does performance management appear to support the strategic commissioning process? Where there is non-alignment, how would you suggest improving it?

References

Allen, B.A., Wade, E. and Dickinson, H. (2009) 'Bridging the divide – commercial procurement and supply chain management: are there lessons for health care commissioning in England?', *Journal of Public Procurement*, vol 9, pp 505-34.

Audit Commission, Care Quality Commission, HM Inspectorate of Constabulary, HM Inspectorate of Prisons, HM Inspectorate of Probation and Ofsted (2010) *One place national overview report*, London: Joint Inspectorates (see authors cited).

Bourgon, J. (ed.) (2011) *A public service renewal agenda for the 21st century: the new synthesis project*, Ottawa: Public Governance International.

Bovaird, T. (2009) *New models of strategic commissioning: report for LGA and CBI*, Birmingham: INLOGOV, University of Birmingham.

Bovaird, T. and Downe, J. (2006) 'N generations of reform: a loosely-coupled armada or ships that pass in the night?', *International Public Management Journal*, vol 9, no 4, pp 429-55.

Bovaird, T. and Loeffler, E. (2011) 'From engagement to co-production: how users and communities coantribute ro public services,' in V. Pestoff, T. Brandsen and B. Verschuere (eds) *New public governance, the third sector and co-production*, London: Routledge.

Bovaird, T., Dickinson, H. and Allen, K. (2010) *Commissioning across government: review of evidence*, Birmingham: Third Sector Research Centre.

Cabinet Office (2006) *Partnership in public services: an action plan for the third sector involvement*, London: Cabinet Office.

Cave, A. (n.d.) *The DWP's commissioning strategy*, available online via: http:// virtual.nationalschool.gov.uk/AJC/Learning%20%20Development/DWP%20 Commissioning%20Strategy.pdf

Commissioning Support Programme (2009) *Achieving better outcomes: commissioning in children's services*, London: Commissioning Support Programme.

DCLG (Department for Communities and Local Government) (2006) *Strong and prosperous communities*, London: TSO.

DCLG (2008) *Strong and prosperous communities: statutory guidance*, London: DCLG.

DCLG (2009a) *Long-term evaluation of LAAs and LSPs: strategic commissioning for place shaping – report of an action learning set*, Warwick: OMP.

DCLG (2009b) *Empowering communities, shaping prospects, transforming life: a vision for intelligent commissioning in local government (informal consultation draft)*, London: DCLG.

DH (Department of Health) (2005) *Independence, well-being and choice: our vision for the future of social care for adults in England*, London: DH.

DH (2006a) *Health reform in England: update and commissioning framework*, London: DH.

DH (2006b) *Our health, our care, our say: a new direction for community services*, London: DH.

DH (2007a) *Commissioning framework for health and well-being*, London: DH.

DH (2007b) *World class commissioning: Vision*, London: DH.

Dickinson, H. (2010) 'The importance of being efficacious: English health and social care partnerships and service user outcomes', PhD thesis, University of Birmingham.

Dickinson, H. and Ham, C. (2008) *The governance of health services in small countries: what are the lessons for Wales?*, Cardiff: NLIAH.

Dixon, J. (1998) 'The context', in J. Le Grand, N. Mays and J. A. Mullidan (eds) *Learning from the NHS internal market: a review of the evidence*, London: King's Fund, pp 1-14.

Ferlie, E., Pettigrew, A., Ashburner, L. and Fitzgerald, L. (1996) *The New Public Management in action*, Oxford: Oxford University Press.

HM Government (2006) *Joint planning and commissioning framework for children, young people and maternity services*, London: Department for Education and Skills and Department of Health.

HM Treasury (2003) *Every child matters*, London: TSO.

Horne, M. and Baeck, P. (2010) *Shaking up commissioning*, London: Innovation Unit and NESTA.

Le Grand, J., Mays, N. and Dixon, J. (1998) 'The reforms: success or failure or neither?', in J. Le Grand, N. Mays and J. A. Mullidan (eds) *Learning from the NHS internal market: a review of the evidence*, London: King's Fund, pp 117-43.

LGA and CBI (Local Government Association and Confederation of British Industry) (2009) *Commissioning strategically for better public services across local government*, London: CBI.

Martin, S., Bovaird, T. and Downe, J. (2009) *Reforming local government: impacts and interactions of central government policies from 2000 to 2006: final report of the meta-evaluation of the local government modernisation agenda*, London: DCLG.

OTS (Office of the Third Sector) (2006) *Partnership in public services*, London: OTS.

Public Administration Select Committee (2008) *Public services and the third sector: rhetoric and reality*, House of Commons, 11th Report of Session 2007-2008, vol 1, London: TSO.

Smith, J. A., Dixon, J., Mays, N., McLeod, H., Goodwin, N., McClelland, S., Lewis, R. and Wyke, S. (2005) 'Practice-based commissioning: applying the evidence, *British Medical Journal*, vol 331, 1397-9.

Vize, R. (2009) 'Andy Burnham speech delivers body blow to NHS competition and choice', *Health Services Journal*, 24 September, www.hsj.co.uk/comment/leader/andy-burnham-speech-delivers-body-blow-to-nhs-competition-and-choice/5006602.article

Walsh, K. (1991) *Competition for local authority services: initial experiences*, London: HMSO.

Walsh, K. and Davis, H. (1993) *Competition and service: the impact of the Local Government Act (1998)*, London: HMSO.

Walters, A. (2009) 'Commissioning: changing the face of local government?', *eGov monitor*, 14 April, www.egovmonitor.com/node/24614

Welsh Assembly Government (2008) *Proposals to change the structure of the NHS in Wales – consultation paper. Proposed new planning system: from a commissioned to a planned system*. Paper 2. Cardiff: Welsh Assembly Government.

Williams, I., Robinson, S. and Dickinson, H. (2011) *Rationing in health care: the theory and practice of priority setting*, Bristol: The Policy Press.

TWO

Needs assessment

Tom Marshall and Eleanor Hothersall

Summary

This chapter explores:

- the importance and nature of needs assessment;
- concepts of need, supply and demand;
- different approaches to/rationales for needs assessment;
- the practical stages involved in a rapid needs assessment.

Needs assessment is an exercise in planning. The purpose of needs assessment is to establish what services or interventions a service ought to provide (see, for example, Stevens and Raferty, 1997). The process by which health and social care practitioners determine the care needs of their individual patients or clients is also referred to as needs assessment. However, this chapter concerns the assessment of need for groups or populations of patients. Why must we undertake needs assessment? The starting point for needs assessment is that there is a mismatch between the services provided and the services we believe ought to be provided. Fundamentally, this is because the factors that determine what services are provided are not the same as the factors that determine what services are needed. Service provision is in large part a reflection of history. The numbers and skill mix of health and social care professionals reflect the numbers who were trained and employed in previous years. Health and social care facilities and the physical infrastructure may reflect decisions taken many decades ago. The services that are provided are therefore driven by past decisions. Alongside this we know that health and social care systems face constant change. The frequency and types of diseases are affected by demographic change. New diseases emerge and others change in frequency. For example, the frequency of chronic diseases is increasing as the population ages and tuberculosis (TB) has increased with increasing migration from high-prevalence countries. We also see changes in healthcare technology. New diagnostic tests may identify more disease or help distinguish between those who should be treated in one way or another. New treatments may replace older treatments, may transform the pattern of a disease (the prognosis of HIV infection is a good example) or may make more patients treatable. In social care, the increasing numbers of older people and people with dementia will mean changes in provision that can be identified and provided for.

A second problem with matching service provision to need is that demand is not simply the sum of individually expressed demands for health and social care. Individual service users are sometimes poor at distinguishing between effective and ineffective care, particularly in a healthcare setting. Therefore, even if services perfectly reflected what patients demanded, they would not reflect what they need (Newhouse, 1993). As health and social care budgets are increasingly personalised, there is a real risk that demand will increase provision of services with little effectiveness (although see Chapters Nine and Eleven, this volume, for an alternative view).

History of needs assessment in the UK

Formal healthcare needs assessment emerged in the National Health Service (NHS) following the NHS and Community Care Act 1990. Prior to this, NHS financial resources were allocated to geographical regions following a resource allocation formula, but less attention was paid to the pattern of services that the resources were used to provide. The allocation of resources was largely based on demography, which was regarded as a proxy for healthcare need (DHSS, 1976). As other chapters in this volume suggest, the NHS and Community Care Act 1990 separated the functions of purchasing and providing healthcare (and, to a certain extent, social care). Organisations that purchase healthcare acquired a responsibility for determining what healthcare they should commission and pay for. Healthcare providers became responsible for meeting the healthcare needs specified by purchasers.

From 1990, responsibility for purchasing healthcare moved from district health authorities, to primary care groups (PCGs) to primary care trusts (PCTs) but remained fundamentally the responsibility of the health service, with a greater or lesser degree of involvement of primary care clinicians. The Local Government and Public Involvement in Health Act 2007 required directors of public health in the health service to collaborate with adult social services and children's services in local government to produce joint strategic needs assessments (JSNAs) for their populations (DCLG, 2008; Ellins and Glasby, 2008). The aim of this is to improve coordination between health services and local authorities and also to consider the wider determinants of health such as housing, employment and the environment – responsibility for which lie outside of the health service. To inform this process, core data on demography, the social environment (deprivation levels), health behaviour, health service use and health outcomes were produced by Public Health Observatories (www.apho.org.uk). Following the 2010 White Paper (DH, 2010), proposals to integrate public health into local government and to emphasise the importance of general practitioner (GP)-led commissioning make such joint working even more important.

—

Supply, demand and need

There are three fundamental definitions that are central to the concept of 'needs assessment' – supply, demand and need:

• By *supply*, we mean the services or treatments that are provided. This means the interventions, drugs or services that are available.
• By *demand*, we mean the services or treatments that service users – or carers acting on their behalf – want. Demand can be expressed, where treatments or services are specifically requested, or demand may be latent. Demand is driven by patients' beliefs about their own state of health, their beliefs or knowledge about what is likely to be beneficial and their awareness of what is available. In the area of health, patients' demand for healthcare is often mediated through a health professional. In the United Kingdom (UK), this is typically a GP. Therefore, a patient's demands for healthcare are mediated to some extent by their GP's beliefs about the patient's health, knowledge about what is effective and awareness of what is available. General practitioners may increase, decrease or alter a patient's demand for healthcare. In a similar way a patient's demand for social care may be mediated by social care professionals, who are a key source of information on what services are available.
• It is common to mistake demand for a health service with need. Patients demand a service when they know the service exists, believe they are likely to benefit from the service and believe the benefits to be greater than the costs of accessing the service. This may be quite unrelated to the service's effectiveness. Similarly, a service that has been used historically may have been superseded or have been found to be ineffective since its inception. In these situations, disinvestment or decommissioning is necessary (see Chapter Five, this volume).
• By *need*, we mean what we believe ought to be provided. Health and social care need is therefore a value judgement about what services ought to be provided. It is worthwhile exploring the philosophies underlying this value judgement in a bit more detail (and we will return to this shortly).

From the three definitions given above, we can see that it is possible to have a situation where there is supply but no need, need but no supply or supply and need but no demand. For example, we might decide that certain patients need influenza immunisation (need) and offer influenza immunisation in primary care (supply) but nobody asks for the service (no demand). The GP might influence demand by actively advising selected patients to have immunisation. Equally, the GP might decide that patients do not need antibiotics for upper respiratory infections (no need) but patients nevertheless ask for antibiotics (demand) and GPs may prescribe them (supply). In prescribing antibiotics, the GP influences this demand by giving the impression to the patient that they should seek antibiotics for the same condition in future, thus contributing to future demand (Little et al, 1997).

Conceptions of need

Since health and social care need is a way of articulating society's views about the services that ought to be provided, we must be able to justify our chosen concept of health and social care need on the basis of its consistency and transparency.

Need as a duty to provide

Different philosophical approaches lead us to different conceptions of need (what we ought to provide). One conception of need is deontological: we have a duty to provide certain services. This may be because there is a legal requirement, because health professionals feel a duty to provide certain services or because there is some other overriding moral imperative to provide the service. If we adopt a deontological approach to needs assessment, when deciding whether there is a need for health and social care the debate focuses on whether there is a legal or ethical imperative to provide the service. Whether the health and social care is effective, whether it serves a useful social objective and whether the benefits are commensurate with the costs are of less concern. Under this conception, need tends to be viewed as an absolute. Either we are obliged to provide a service or we are not.

This conception of need is most clear in a contractual situation such as health insurance. If the health insurance policy specifies that a service is not covered, there is no obligation to supply it. Examples of this way of thinking about healthcare need are found to some extent in the UK NHS. For example, ambulances are obliged to bring patients to hospital if they request it. Health professionals sometimes feel obliged to treat certain patients irrespective of whether the patients will benefit from treatment. Other required rules include an obligation to see referred patients (or service users in social care) or an obligation to carry out elective surgery within a specified period of time.

The deontological approach is rule based. Since it is impossible to write rules to cover every conceivable situation, this approach is not helpful for the unclear decisions required in most circumstances. Such a sweeping approach can also have cost implications.

Need as determined by health or social care professionals

Health and social care needs require a problem to be accepted as a health or social care problem. Since health and social care professionals are responsible for defining health/social care problems, they also define the limits of health/social care need. For example, if prevailing medical opinion redefines a condition as a variation of normality rather than an illness (for example sexual orientation), treatment is no longer a healthcare need. Most individuals or families take care of their own care needs. Therefore, for there to be a social care need, professionals must agree that the person's care needs are of a magnitude or character to require society's intervention.

Need as capacity to benefit

A third interpretation of healthcare need is utilitarian (or consequentialist). Here, we distinguish between 'neediness' and 'need for'. Those in poor health need better health. Poor health can be described by looking at the frequency of disease. But need-for-health or 'neediness' is distinct from need for healthcare. Poor health only generates a need for health services to the extent that health services can improve health. By this definition of healthcare need there is a healthcare need because we have evidence that a service is effective at reasonable cost. In other words, the need for care is related to the likely consequences of providing that care. Debates about this kind of need focus on evidence of the health effects and sometimes wider social effects of health and social care and the cost. Under this conception, all needs are viewed as relative (see Chapter Three, this volume, for more on prioritisation). Any service that can provide any health benefit at any cost can be considered to represent a potential need. The main consideration is one of relative priority, whether there is a greater reason to provide one service or another. Those services that offer the greatest potential to improve health are those that are most needed. The aim of needs assessment is to provide the greatest benefit within available resources, whether the focus is on health or social care, or a combination of the two.

Needs assessment based on capacity to benefit requires a method for measuring health benefit. First, we need to ask what benefits we are interested in and from whose perspective. When we restore health there are also wider societal benefits resulting from restoring patients to full productivity. Including these wider societal benefits would mean that we must assess patients' productivity value to society. This approach would give greater weight to those in more skilled, more valued occupations (such as skilled professionals). But this runs against the equity principles of the NHS. In some circumstances one person's health is influenced by that of another. For example, if we treat TB we also prevent others from contracting TB. Were we to ignore such health benefits we would underestimate the benefits of treating infectious diseases, therefore we normally include health benefits to others that are the result of infectious diseases. A more complex question is whether we should include health (or non-health) benefits to others, which result from treating non-infectious diseases. For example, if we provide services for patients with dementia, there may be little health benefit for the patient but substantial health (or non-health) benefit to their carers. Failing to include such health benefits may underestimate the wider benefits of providing care for such patients. But if we do this for dementia, we should also do so for other conditions where carers are substantially involved. The key is to be consistent when considering health benefits (see Box 2.1 for an example).

Box 2.1: Anti-dementia drugs: a case study

In 2001, the National Institute for Health and Clinical Excellence (NICE) published guidance on the use of drugs (donepezil, galantamine and rivastigmine) licensed for the treatment of dementia (NICE, 2001). Despite initial media hype, the drug was not a 'cure' for dementia, and the original drug trials probably overstated the efficacy of the medication (Melzer, 1998). NICE's economic model showed cost-effectiveness only for 'moderate dementia', and consequently this was the only clinical situation in which NICE would approve the use of these drugs. The drug manufacturers and charities involved with dementia care argued that this economic model was flawed, in part because it failed to take into account the improvement in quality of life for carers that the medication provided. As mentioned above, this argument posed a considerable challenge to NICE, since considering the perspective of the carer in one condition was likely to require similar considerations in the future. In 2007, following judicial review, NICE was forced to provide the drug companies with the economic model it used, and subsequently revised its guidelines in light of the drug companies' comments (NICE, 2007). This time it did indeed consider the impact on carers in addition to the patients themselves. The altered model did not, however, affect the final recommendations and at present these drugs are still limited to use in moderate dementia.

Interestingly, the most recent draft guidance on the treatment of dementia (http://guidance. nice.org.uk/TA/WaveR111/1) now indicates that the evidence is strong enough for these drugs to be used in mild dementia.

Rationale for need as capacity to benefit

The rationale for using the concept of capacity to benefit as a definition of need is as follows. UK health and social care is funded from public resources. Needs assessment is therefore fundamentally concerned with allocating public resources. It follows that those resources should be allocated in a way that is transparent and which can be rationally justified as meeting the public's needs. Since capacity to benefit includes the whole public, a method of resource allocation that maximises capacity to benefit is by definition the best use of those resources (discussed in Chapter Three). Using reproducible scientific evidence to justify decisions means that the process is both transparent and rational.

Need and equity

Equity is a principle of distributional justice, which is a further factor to be considered in relation to health and social care need. In other words, we are not only concerned with providing health and social care services, we also are concerned with who gets what. This means that we give greater weight to meeting health and social care needs in one group than another. There are many principles of distributional justice and in theory we could prioritise groups by any chosen method and describe this as equitable in accordance with our chosen version of equity. For example, in a private health insurance system, it is a legal principle that healthcare benefits are only offered to those who have paid for insurance.

One superficially attractive idea in a publicly funded system is to give lower weight to meeting the healthcare needs of those who bear a degree of responsibility for causing their illness ('desert' – see Chapter Three). However, this raises many problems. We must decide when an individual is responsible for their actions. Are smokers responsible for their own lung cancer? Many smokers took up the habit as children and quitting is difficult. Are they just as responsible as those who took up smoking in adulthood? And most smokers do not suffer from lung cancer, but can suffer from other unrelated illnesses. In effect, by singling out those smokers who are unlucky enough to develop smoking-related illnesses, we are arbitrarily selecting out some smokers to be low priority while others are not. What about the consumption of a Western diet? Should UK citizens who consume a traditional British diet be a lower priority for treatment of heart disease than those who consume a Mediterranean diet? The ethical basis for dividing the ill into the deserving and undeserving may be debatable (Loughlin, 2002), but the practical application of such a rule is not: it is an arbitrary and impractical approach to prioritisation.

Because the founding principles of the NHS were to address access to healthcare by more socially deprived groups, in the UK we interpret equity as meaning that we give greater weight (or at least no less weight) to individuals from socially disadvantaged groups. The main practical questions that face us are therefore the criteria for considering an individual to belong to a socially disadvantaged population. In other words, we must think about equity in relation to:

- age;
- gender;
- ethnicity (for example majority versus minority ethnic group);
- geography (for example urban versus rural);
- socioeconomics status (for example less affluent versus more affluent).

In some cases we might consider equity in relation to other characteristics such as religious affiliation or sexuality (indeed, it is a legal requirement).

Key evidence in needs assessment

Health benefit

Because we are using public resources to improve the public's health, we must measure health in a way that is meaningful to the public. This means improvement in quality of life, improvement in function and improvement in length of life. Changes in clinical parameters alone do not represent improvements in health unless there are good grounds to indicate that they are likely to lead to improvement in quality, function or length of life. When determining which of two interventions for the same condition produces the greatest health benefit, this is relatively straightforward. We can measure the number of patients restored to full health (or whose condition improved) using a disease-specific measurement. However, when comparing conditions that are different, we need a measure of generic improvements in health. The quality-adjusted life year (QALY) is one generic measure of health that encompasses quality of life and length of life (see Box 2.2; see also Chapter Three, this volume, for further discussion).

Box 2.2: The quality-adjusted life year (QALY)

Although it is beyond the scope of this chapter to describe the derivation of a QALY, it is necessary to understand what a QALY is intended to indicate. A year of full health is given a value of 1 and being dead is given a value of 0. Health states of less than full health are given values between 0 and 1. These values are derived from a population survey and are therefore taken to be indicative of the public's valuation of health states. The values are preference based. This means that members of the public were asked to indicate whether they prefer a lower risk of death (or a greater length of life) in a poor health state or a higher risk of death (or a shorter length of life) in full health. At the point at which individuals cannot decide between the two alternatives, they are considered of equal value.

For example, imagine I cannot choose between being in health state A for 10 years or a gamble of a 50% chance of death with a 50% chance of full health. This implies that I value five years of full health the same as 10 years of health state A. Therefore, each year of health state A has a QALY value of 0.5. A drug that effected a year's cure of this health state would therefore achieve a health gain of 0.5 QALYs.

Evidence of benefit

When examining health benefit, we consider the familiar hierarchy of evidence. The strongest evidence is based on systematic reviews of randomised controlled trials, followed by single randomised controlled trials, cohort studies, case series, theory-based conjecture and expert opinion. Greater weight should be given to stronger evidence (although see Glasby, 2011, for an alternative view and a discussion of broader concepts of 'knowledge-based practice'). This is much more difficult in social care, where interventions are generally much less subject to rigorous evaluation. Where such evaluations have taken place they have tended to focus on technological developments (such as telecare or telehealth; see Ekeland et al, 2010) or on areas of mental health (Evers et al, 2007). Carer burden is measured within these settings (Dixon et al, 2006), but it is hard to see how this could be extrapolated to other social care settings.

—

Measurement of resource costs

Resource costs include capital costs, consumables and productive time (generally staff costs). It is possible to assess costs from a societal perspective, a government perspective or a health service perspective. In healthcare commissioning until recently, most commonly we assessed costs from a health service perspective, where shifting costs from the NHS to social services or to informal carers was therefore seen as a reduction in costs. As more commissioning for health and social care is joint or comes to rest at a local authority level, the true costs will be more apparent (see also Chapter Ten, this volume).

Undertaking a needs assessment

There are three main ways to undertake healthcare needs assessment:

- epidemiological needs assessment;
- corporate needs assessment;
- comparative needs assessment.

The main method is epidemiological needs assessment but corporate and comparative needs assessments may be carried out as part of a wider needs assessment. These are described in more detail below as part of the process of undertaking a needs assessment.

Epidemiological needs assessment

This is a comprehensive approach to needs assessment. In this approach, the frequency of the health problem is described, the interventions that are effective are identified and current services in relation to these effective interventions are mapped. The aim of the needs assessment is to identify which gaps between current services and the most effective services should be prioritised for service change. Before initiating a needs assessment, the terms of reference must be clear. A needs assessment starts with a health problem (for example what services should we provide for adult diabetics?), not with a service (for example how many specialist diabetic nurses should we employ?). It must be clear which health problems the needs assessment is to address; and which health problems it is not to address.

In almost every case when one organisation carries out a healthcare needs assessment, another organisation has already completed a similar exercise. It is essential to make contact with other public health specialists, health and social commissioners or agencies to ask their advice and to make use of their work. This is best done through electronic mailing lists such as JISCMAIL (www.jiscmail. ac.uk). A further valuable resource is the collection of healthcare needs assessments that are held online at the University of Birmingham (www.hcna.bham.ac.uk).

Healthcare needs assessment is normally carried out by a team. This should include relevant health professionals from primary care, secondary care and specialist care. There is a need for some public health or epidemiological expertise. If possible, patients or carers should be represented. In addition, the team may need to liaise with other individuals or departments to provide supplementary information (see Box 2.3).

Box 2.3: Members of a healthcare needs assessment team

- Primary care health professionals (doctors and/or nursing staff)
- Public health specialist
- Other relevant professionals (for example professions allied to medicine)
- Secondary care specialists (for example nurse specialists or consultants)
- Patient representatives (lay board members, patient groups)
- Other relevant agencies (social services, housing, voluntary groups).

Corporate needs assessment

This is a rapid appraisal of healthcare needs by a group representing the key stakeholders such as the healthcare needs assessment team. Stakeholders outline the key effective services and the extent to which there are enough of each of these services. Services can then be prioritised according to the gap between potential effectiveness and service availability.

The advantages of this approach are that it is rapid and that it engages the key stakeholders. It can help establish if there are any services there is an absolute legal or ethical duty to provide. Similarly, it can establish whether there are any areas that fall outside of the health arena and therefore need not be considered. The main disadvantage is that stakeholders tend to see healthcare needs through the prism of existing services and this can mean that they assess demand rather than need. However, there are more systematic approaches to undertaking corporate needs assessment, such as programme budgeting and marginal analysis (PBMA) (Ruta et al, 2005; see also Chapter Three, this volume).

This is a pragmatic method for undertaking a corporate needs assessment. It is essentially a method for allocating financial resources between health services. For each disease-related programme under consideration, the amount of financial resources that are available is first established. Second, where these resources are currently being spent is established. For example what resources are allocated to diabetes care? How much is spent on prevention, primary care and secondary care? Of primary care spending, how much is spent on drugs, diagnostics, staff and so on? Third, these resources are related to health benefits. How much benefit results from primary care compared to secondary care? Two questions are then asked: if more resources were made available, what would be the best way to spend those resources in order to achieve the most health gain? If fewer resources were available, where could spending be cut with the least effect on health gain? If the stakeholders judge the gains to one programme from increased funding to be greater than the losses to another programme from reduced funding, then some of the funding should be moved from one service to another where it will have greater benefit. The process is repeated in subsequent years until movement of funding will not produce greater benefit through further redistribution. Programme budgeting requires financial information about which resources are being used for which types of clinical conditions. This may be hard to obtain because staff work across more than one clinical area and facilities are used by more than one type of patient. However, to facilitate the process, programme budgets have been produced by the NHS Information Centre (www.nchod. nhs.uk/). These allow users to see expenditure on specific disease groups within defined geographical regions. The expenditure can be related to health service use or health outcomes.

Comparative needs assessment

This is another rapid method of needs assessment. Essentially, it means comparing service provision, service use or health outcomes between different geographical areas. For the purposes of comparison, these figures should be standardised to take account of demographic differences between populations. Service provision means the capacity of facilities or numbers of staff; service use means numbers of consultations, prescriptions issued, diagnostic tests performed or procedures carried out; health outcome means frequency of disease or mortality. There is always some variation in standardised rates of service provision, service use or health outcomes, but this should be consistent with chance. Large variations in service use or service provision merit further investigation. The underlying assumption is that unusual variation in services represents either over-provision or under-provision and can be used as a guide to where services should be increased or decreased.

Comparative needs assessment is quick to carry out. It can be useful for assessing equity in service provision, service use or even outcomes in different population groups. However, it is constrained by the availability of comparative data and it assumes that health service provision *somewhere* is at the right level. Data sources for comparative needs assessment may be obtained from primary care, secondary care or from specific research. Primary care data from the Quality and Outcomes Framework (QOF) can give an indication of the prevalence of known chronic diseases such as coronary heart disease or asthma (www.qof.ic.nhs.uk/).

Different stages

When conducting a more rapid needs assessment, there are typically six steps – each of which is set out below (see Figure 2.1; see also Box 2.4, page 58, for a practical case study).

Figure 2.1: The healthcare needs assessment process

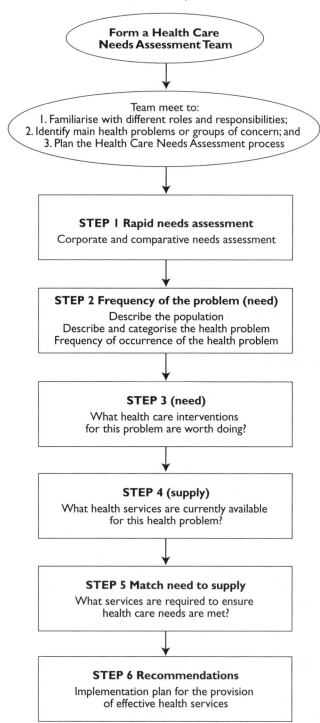

Step 1: Rapid needs assessment

Realistically, there are times when the only feasible needs assessment is the quickest one possible. In these situations, it is vital that the information collected is as accurate and useful as possible.

Step 2: Determine the frequency of the health problem (need)

The aim of this step is to estimate the burden of disease. By this we mean the number of occurrences of the disease or health problem in the population. For acute problems with short-term implications (such as accidents), this is the incidence multiplied by the relevant population. For chronic problems with long-term health implications (such as diabetes), the more relevant measure is the prevalence of the problem.

Describing the population

Demography determines the frequency of most diseases. It is therefore usually necessary to describe the characteristics of the population of concern. In particular, this means the age-sex structure but it may also include ethnicity or deprivation levels if these are important determinants of disease frequency (for example for diabetes or coronary heart disease). For planning into the future we need to know how the population is likely to change in the next few years. These data are available from the Office for National Statistics (www.statistics.gov.uk).

Describing and categorising the health problem

At this stage we also need to describe the frequency (incidence for acute illness, prevalence for chronic illness) of the health problem in relation to the population of interest.

Most health problems have important variations in severity and treatment. The health problem should therefore be divided into relevant subcategories, which may be dealt with separately. For example, back pain is categorised by the presence or absence of serious underlying disease. Back pain without underlying disease can be further subcategorised into new episodes, recurrent episodes, persistent episodes and chronic back pain. Each of these requires a different intervention.

Sources of information

The most accurate information on incidence or prevalence of a disease comes from epidemiological studies. Such studies use standard case definitions and assess entire populations, providing a numerator (cases of disease) and a denominator (total population).

Cancer registries provide information on the frequency of cancers, which is of a similar quality to research studies (www.ukacr.org/).

Electronic primary care records can provide estimates of incidence or prevalence. This is because they have a numerator (cases of disease) and a denominator (the total registered population). However, these are estimates of recorded incidence. Data derived from electronic primary care records often underestimate prevalence or incidence because of under-reporting or under-diagnosis. They may also overestimate prevalence or incidence because of under-reporting or misdiagnosis. It is always helpful to compare figures derived from routine data sources with epidemiological data in order to determine the likely direction and extent of error.

Hospital data can also provide information on frequency of disease or service use (www.hesonline.nhs.uk/). One problem with these data is that while the numerator (cases of disease, hospital episodes) may be well defined, the denominator (the total population of concern) may be unclear if the hospital does not have a stable and well-defined catchment area.

Bespoke data collection

It is possible to conduct local surveys of disease frequency for needs assessment. However, this should only be resorted to when there are no alternative data sources. Conducting surveys is time consuming and expensive. If not carried out by epidemiological researchers they are prone to bias and producing inaccurate results. Finally, the precision of results obtained from a small local survey is rarely sufficient to provide a different answer to that obtained by applying epidemiological data from another setting.

Step 3: Describe the effective and cost-effective interventions (need)

The next step is to identify the services and interventions that are effective for the health problem under consideration. In many cases, work has already been undertaken to appraise evidence of effectiveness and to define which services should be provided.

The key data sources for this include NICE (www.nice.org.uk) and the Scottish Intercollegiate Guidelines Network (SIGN; www.sign.ac.uk). This is because these bodies base their guidance on systematic appraisal of evidence of effectiveness and cost-effectiveness. Where UK guidelines are not available there may be guidelines from other countries that follow similar transparent processes and base their recommendations on appraised evidence of effectiveness and cost-effectiveness.

Professional bodies often also produce guidelines, but the processes by which they reach their recommendations may not be as clear. Some guidelines may be little more than advocacy for sufferers of a specific disease or for a specific health service intervention.

If evidence-based guidelines are not available, evidence of effectiveness can be sought (Iqbal et al, 2006). This follows the hierarchy described earlier, with greatest weight given to systematic reviews of randomised controlled trials (for example, Cochrane reviews, NICE reviews), followed by single randomised controlled trials, cohort studies and so on (but see the comments earlier regarding evidence in social care).

It may help to draw up a table, listing the health problems being considered (in one column) alongside interventions (in the next column) and evidence of effectiveness (in a third column). It is also important to record when there is no evidence and when there is evidence that services are ineffective.

Step 4: Describe the services that are currently provided (supply)

A description of current services is necessarily very specific to the population of concern. This part of the process is likely to be led by those involved in service provision and by patient or carer representatives This should include the full range from highly specialised care to primary care. In some cases it will include voluntary sector services, other government services (for example social services) and various kinds of informal and self-care (such as access to appropriate information and over-the-counter medication). It may also include prevention or health promotion activities that are related to the service of interest, for example smoking cessation in relation to coronary heart disease. It is also important to describe the pathways by which patients or service users access care. This should describe where patients first make contact with the relevant services and how they are referred on to other services. This may be best described using a flow diagram.

Step 5: Match need to supply

The next stage in the process is to identify gaps in provision. Are there evidence-based and cost-effective interventions that are under-provided? Are interventions that are not evidence based or cost-effective provided? Where are the greatest gains likely to be achieved at least resource cost? Are there areas suitable for disinvestment?

Step 6: Recommendations and implementation plan

The final step in the process is to make recommendations for changes to meet the prioritised gaps in need. This should involve practical steps towards implementation.

Box 2.4: Case study: kidney disease

A healthcare needs assessment team for renal disease should consist of at least one specialist renal clinician, at least one primary care clinician, a representative of patients with renal disease and a public health specialist. The health problem can be categorised as prevention of renal disease in the population at risk (diabetics, hypertensives and those with acute kidney disease); management of early renal disease; and management of renal failure disease requiring dialysis. Classification of kidney disease by severity may be helpful when estimating the frequency of disease.

Rapid needs assessment

The key stakeholders can undertake a corporate needs assessment. One difficulty with this approach will be that patients with dialysis needs are highly visible whereas those with untreated kidney failure in the community may be invisible and uncounted.

The Public Health Observatories have produced extensive data on kidney disease for all English PCTs (www.erpho.org.uk/). These include the frequency of recorded kidney failure in primary care (from the QOF); the standardised mortality rate from chronic renal failure; and spending on renal disease compared to need. This allows for rapid comparative needs assessment to be undertaken. It is likely to be agreed that for kidney disease there is an overriding ethical duty to treat patients with kidney failure who need dialysis.

Determine the frequency of the health problem (need)

Figures on the expected prevalence of renal disease and renal failure can be obtained from Public Health Observatories. This can be compared to the prevalence of diagnosed renal disease as described in QOF data.

Describe the effective and cost-effective interventions (need)

There are NICE and SIGN guidelines on the management of kidney disease. These would be a key source for defining which services are effective for the prevention and management of kidney disease (www.nice.org.uk/CG73 and www.sign.ac.uk/guidelines/fulltext/103/index. html). Effective treatments include dietary interventions, smoking cessation advice, blood pressure control, use of ACE inhibitors and ARB 2 blockers, and management of diabetes. Key questions of cost-effectiveness for the management of those with renal failure are the relative cost-effectiveness of hospital-based dialysis, home dialysis and renal transplantation. Patients' views on these treatment options are also important in determining relative priorities.

Describe the services that are currently provided (supply)

The healthcare needs assessment team must provide information on the facilities and staff available in primary and secondary care for the management of renal disease. Some information on spending is available from the Public Health Observatories. Particular attention should be paid to the pathways to care followed by patients. This means the way in which kidney disease is detected and managed in primary care; referral pathways to specialist care; and access to specialist centres for renal transplantation. The proportions of patients managed by hospital dialysis, home dialysis and renal transplantation are likely to be important since these treatments differ in their cost-effectiveness. Given that renal disease is more frequent in populations with a high prevalence of diabetes (particularly South Asians), equity of access to and use by these populations is also an important consideration.

Match need to supply

The relationship between existing services and services that are known to be effective needs to be mapped out. Under-provided but cost-effective services should be identified and any over-provided but less cost-effective services also identified. Recommendations will need to be made to address the unmet need.

Summary

Healthcare needs assessment is a process for deciding what services ought to be provided. It is therefore an exercise in rational planning. Needs assessment is driven by an underlying philosophy. The most practical philosophical approach is utilitarian. This takes the view that since the purpose of healthcare is to achieve improvements in health, the fundamental aim of healthcare needs assessment should be to identify services that are effective at improving health and prioritise them in relation to their efficiency at improving health. There is an important distinction between services that patients demand and services for which there is evidence of effectiveness. Fundamentally, the extent of healthcare need is determined by the effectiveness of the intervention, not by the scale of the problem.

In practical terms, the process of undertaking a healthcare needs assessment can be divided into three related exercises. The first is to determine the size of the health problem by establishing how frequently people suffer from the illness in question. This requires epidemiological data. The second is to determine the effectiveness and cost-effectiveness of interventions to deal with the problem. This requires evidence of effectiveness. The third is to determine the services that are already provided for the problem. This requires local knowledge. The practical implementation of a needs assessment is a planned and prioritised series of steps to change the services that are provided so that they are more closely aligned with evidence of effectiveness and cost-effectiveness.

Further reading

A series of articles in the *British Medical Journal* describes approaches to health needs assessment:

- Jordan, J., Dowsell, T., Harrison, S., Lilford, L. J. and Mort, M. (1998) 'Whose priorities? Listening to users and the public', *British Medical Journal*, vol 316, pp 1668-70.

- Stevens, A. and Gillam, S. (1998) 'Needs assessment: from theory to practice', *British Medical Journal*, vol 316, pp 1448-52.
- Wilkinson, J. R. and Murray, S. A. (1998) 'Assessment in primary care: practical issues and possible approaches', *British Medical Journal*, vol 316, p 1524.
- Williams, R. and Wright, J. (1998) 'Epidemiological issues in health needs assessment', *British Medical Journal*, vol 316, pp 1379-82.
- Wright, J., Williams, R. and Wilkinson, J.R. (1998) 'Development and importance of health needs assessment', *British Medical Journal*, vol 316, pp 1310-13.

Other key sources include Stevens, A., Raftery, J., Mant, J. and Simspon, S. (eds) (2004) *Health care needs assessment*, vols 1 and 2, Oxford: Radcliffe Publishing. These books are the 'bible' of epidemiologically based healthcare needs assessment and invaluable resources. They contain chapters covering a number of epidemiologically based key healthcare needs assessments and a template for how to approach a needs assessment in a systematic way. They are also available online (see below). For further discussion of priority setting and rationing, see Chapter Three, this volume, by Williams and Robinson, as well as Williams, I., Robinson, S. and Dickinson, H. (2011) *Rationing in health care: the theory and practice of priority setting*, Bristol: The Policy Press.

Useful websites

- University of Birmingham Health Care Needs Assessment: www.hcna.bham. ac.uk. This is an online version of the Health Care Needs Assessment series. It includes a large number of epidemiological healthcare needs assessments and is both an invaluable source of information and a template for healthcare needs assessment.
- The NHS Information Centre: Clinical and Health Outcomes Knowledge Base (www.nchod.nhs.uk/), QOF (www.qof.ic.nhs.uk/) and Hospital Episode Statistics Online (www.hesonline.nhs.uk/). The NHS Information Centre is a key source of information on effectiveness (Clinical and Health Outcomes Knowledge Base), prevalence in primary care (QOF) and hospital activity (Hospital Episode Statistics). The first of these is a source of information on services that should be provided. The last two are indications of services provided in primary and secondary care
- National Institute for Health and Clinical Excellence (NICE): www.nice.org. uk/ and Scottish Intercollegiate Guidelines Network (SIGN): www.sign.ac.uk/. NICE and SIGN are essential sources of information on the effectiveness of interventions. They are therefore a guide as to what services should be provided.
- JISCMAIL (www.jiscmail.ac.uk/). JISCMAIL hosts a number of emailing lists. These are essential for anyone undertaking a needs assessment who would like to share best practice and make use of work carried out in other parts of the UK.

- Joint strategic needs assessment (JSNA) guidance: www.dh.gov.uk/en/ Publicationsandstatistics/Publications/PublicationsPolicyAndGuidance/ DH_081097
- The Association of Public Health Observatories: www.apho.org.uk/default. aspx. This includes a wide range of information on the prevalence of diseases, spending and services provided.

Reflective exercises

1. How would you explain to the media or to the general public that a service that was demanded was not needed?
2. Can you identify situations where consideration of costs from an NHS perspective alone may make an important difference to the apparent costs of a service? How could this affect the prioritisation of healthcare needs?
3. Can you identify situations where consideration of health benefits only to the patient may make an important difference to the effectiveness of a service? How could this affect the prioritisation of healthcare needs?
4. List a number of disadvantages of relying on professional experts for information about healthcare needs.

References

DCLG (Department for Communities and Local Government) (2008) *Creating strong, safe and prosperous local communities*, London: TSO.

DH (Department of Health) (2010) *Equity and excellence: liberating the NHS*, www.dh.gov.uk/en/Publicationsandstatistics/Publications/ PublicationsPolicyAndGuidance/DH_117353

DHSS (Department of Health and Social Security) (1976) *Sharing resources for health in England: report of the Resource Allocation Working Party*, London: DHSS.

Dixon, S., Walker, M. and Salek, S. (2006) 'Incorporating carer effects into economic evaluation', *PharmacoEconomics*, vol 24, no 1, pp 43-53.

Ekeland, A. G., Bowes, A. and Flottorp, S. (2010) 'Effectiveness of telemedicine: a systematic review of reviews', *International Journal of Medical Informatics*, vol 79, no 11, pp 736-71.

Ellins, J. and Glasby, J. (2008) *Implementing joint strategic needs assessment: pitfalls, possibilities and progress*, Birmingham: Health Services Management Centre and Department of Health.

Evers, S., Salvador-Curulla, L., Halsteinli, V., McDavid, D. and the MHEEN Group (2007) 'Implementing mental health economic evaluation evidence: building a bridge between theory and practice', *Journal of Mental Health*, vol 16, no 2, pp 223-41.

Glasby, J. (ed) (2011) *Evidence, policy and practice: critical perspectives in health and social care*, Bristol: The Policy Press.

Iqbal, Z., Pryce, A. and Afza, M. (2006) 'Rationalizing rationing in health care: experience of two primary care trusts', *Journal of Public Health*, vol 28, no 2, pp 125-32.

Little, P. S., Gould, C., Williamson, I., Warner, G., Gantley, M. and Kinmonth, A. K. (1997) 'Reattendance and complications in a randomised trial of prescribing strategies for sore throat: the medicalising effect of prescribing antibiotics', *British Medical Journal*, vol 315, pp 350-2.

Loughlin, M. (2002) *Ethics, management and mythology: rational decision making for health service professionals*, Abingdon: Radcliffe Medical Press.

Melzer, D. (1998) 'New drug treatment for Alzheimer's disease: lessons for healthcare policy', *British Medical Journal*, vol 316, p 762.

Newhouse, J. P. (1993) *Free for all? Lessons from the Rand Health Insurance Experiment*, Cambridge, MA: Harvard University Press.

NICE (National Institute for Health and Clinical Excellence) (2001) *Alzheimer's disease (mild to moderate) – donepezil, rivastigmine and galantamine technology appraisal TA19*, http://guidance.nice.org.uk/TA19

NICE (2007) *Donepezil, galantamine, rivastigmine (review) and memantine for the treatment of Alzheimer's disease technology appraisal TA111*, http://guidance.nice.org.uk/TA111/Guidance/Evidence

Ruta, D., Mitton, C., Bate, A. and Donaldson, C. (2005) 'Programme budgeting and marginal analysis: bridging the divide between doctors and managers', *British Medical Journal*, vol 330, pp 1501-3.

Stevens, A. and Raferty, J. (eds) (1997) *Health care needs assessment* (second series), Oxford: Radcliffe Medical Press.

THREE

Decision making and priority setting

Iestyn Williams and Suzanne Robinson

Summary

This chapter explores:
- key features of resource allocation/priority setting in English health and social care;
- ethical principles and public involvement in priority setting;
- evidence and decision making (including key economic approaches);
- issues of politics and accountability.

Introduction

The need to limit the supply of potentially beneficial services and interventions has existed since the early years of the welfare state and, despite recent investment, remains stubbornly in place. In healthcare in particular, this creates huge tensions for those discharging budgets, as principles of universality and comprehensiveness are inevitably compromised. Although the nature of priority setting decisions, and their implementation, vary across countries and over time, the *inevitability* of setting limits on healthcare provision – and therefore the need to create transparent and fair processes for doing so – has become increasingly accepted (Coast, 2004; Newdick, 2005). Furthermore, the importance of the priority-setting agenda increases in times of economic downturn, with the public sector facing severe funding constraints following years of incremental (and, in the case of health in the United Kingdom [UK], substantial) resource growth. Although curbing escalating costs of health and social care has been a preoccupation of nation states for decades, the imperative to distribute scarce resources in an efficient and effective manner has therefore been given extra urgency in recent times. These aspects of the political and economic context underline the importance of priority setting as a component of effective commissioning.

Any expanded definition of health and social care commissioning – such as that adopted in this text – is therefore likely to include priority setting. However, just as there is more to commissioning than making resource allocation decisions, priority setting also cannot be reduced to the commissioning function. Priority-setting decisions are also taken by, for example, provider organisations through formulary lists, assessment and eligibility regimes, medicines management and so on, and by other bodies discharging health and social care budgets. As well as being a widely distributed task, priority setting also contains a number of elements that are not necessarily related to decision making. These aspects include entering into dialogue with external stakeholders (including government, interest groups and the public) and the complex business of the implementation of priority-setting decisions. So although commissioners are invariably expected to carry out priority setting, they are rarely in a position to take full responsibility for all of its dimensions. Clearly, the main focus of this chapter is on those elements of priority setting that are most obviously connected to the commissioning function in publicly funded systems. However, the responsibilities of other parties – for example government, service users and providers, citizens and other stakeholders – are also discussed in order that the relationship of these parties to the commissioning function can be examined. Therefore, the aims of this chapter are to explore the purposes of priority setting and the barriers to achieving these, as well as to put forward some possible solutions for those operating with these difficult briefs. The discussion draws on existing theories, practice and evidence from a wide range of disciplines to outline and explore the operationalisation of priority setting in health and social care (see Williams et al, 2011, for further discussion of these issues).

Health and social care settings

The entire rationing enterprise is predicated on the assumption that public resources are finite and therefore that choices between potentially beneficial areas of investment must be made. The allocation of health and social care resources typically has a number of decision points, including: the setting of overall budgets; distributing resources across services areas, interventions and service user groups; and decisions made by or on behalf of individual patients and service users. Assuming that demand for care outstrips capacity for its provision, these decisions can be understood as a form of resource *rationing*. Over the last few decades, a considerable literature has developed in relation to rationing of healthcare. In particular, there has been much debate over how to make fair population-based decisions over the allocation of resources. This proactive approach is usually referred to as *priority setting* (or prioritisation), which is defined as the setting of rules, processes and criteria for restricting access to care on grounds of cost. This definition excludes the informal and implicit 'bedside' rationing that has traditionally been a feature of healthcare systems (Mechanic, 1995; Klein et al, 1996).

Despite persistent concerns at the extent to which rationing can ever become fully explicit (see, for example, Mechanic, 1995; Coast, 1997), there has been an undeniable, international shift towards the development of formal criteria and processes for setting priorities and making resource allocation decisions. However, social care remains largely absent from these developments and therefore does not feature as explicitly in descriptions of the commissioning role. We might postulate a number of possible reasons for this. First, healthcare tends to occupy a higher-profile and higher-status position within the collective consciousness of societies. The centrality of good health to human life has, for example, led some commentators to postulate it to be a 'special good' worthy of exceptional consideration among public sector priorities (Mooney, 1998). Irrespective of the validity of such claims, there is some support for the notion that healthcare (along with education) ranks high in the order of public sector functions. As a national institution, the National Health Service (NHS), for example, is expected to demonstrate excellence, fairness and comprehensiveness across the country. By comparison, the organisation and delivery of social services are less well known or understood by the general public. Indeed, public pressure is more likely to be towards *reductions* in expenditure on social care than it is to increases (Bergmark, 1996). Arguably, this leads to a level of societal, as well as interest-group, pressure to improve healthcare services not seen in relation to social care (and other public provision). Furthermore, the cost pressures created by advances in medical technology and the proliferation of expensive pharmaceutical interventions outstrip anything seen in the social care arena – although here too there are significant cost pressures.

As well as these factors, there is often considerable divergence between health and social care in terms of funding, decision-making and accountability structures. This is especially marked in England where social care is funded and administered by local (as opposed to national) government and means testing is employed. This has enabled different strategies for rationing resources than the explicit decision making advocated in much of the health-related priority-setting literature. In social care, less responsibility for the setting of priorities resides with commissioners. Instead, the primary means of rationing resources are individual assessment and eligibility criteria and, increasingly, the service user as rationing agent discharging their own individual budgets (see Chapter Eleven, this volume). The traditional role of the public sector population-based decision maker has thus diminished (Scourfield, 2007). We recommend that more work is done to identify and critique the resource allocation mechanisms in social care in terms of the major themes discussed here: namely evidence, ethics, processes, politics and involvement. Equally, if joint commissioning is to be effective (see Chapter Ten, this volume), priority setting will need to take place as part of this broader commissioning mandate. For the purposes of this chapter, however, we are confined by the paucity of evidence and literature and therefore focus primarily on priority setting in healthcare.

Although priority setting takes place in every healthcare system, the mechanisms can vary according to context. For example, heavily centralised systems create a stronger hand for governments to set the 'basket' of reimbursed treatments, whereas local decision makers have more discretion in systems marked by devolution of decision making. Although many countries have been required to separate purchasing from provision of healthcare, much variation exists in the ways in which this has been implemented. For example, tax-based systems differ markedly from those funded out of insurance (either private or social) in which third-party payers play an important role in the rationing of resources. Following recent reform of the English NHS, primary care trusts (PCTs) have emerged as the principal agent of resource allocation (Russell and Greenhalgh, 2009) – although this is now changing again following the election of a new government. In order to demonstrate 'world class' performance, PCTs have previously sought to excel in relation to a number of competencies (DH, 2008), two of which relate specifically to priority setting: the requirement to demonstrate an evidence-based approach to investment decision making and the imperative to deliver efficiency and value for money across healthcare spend. Towards these ends, PCTs have been charged with: overall budget allocation; reprioritising across programme budget areas; disease/care pathway redesign; and substitution of, and disinvestment in, interventions and services. However, with the new government's announcement that PCTs are to be phased out in favour of clinician-based commissioning, there remains doubt over whether and to what extent these competencies will retain their status (Cabinet Office, 2010). What is clear, however, is that the need to use scarce resources efficiently remains, and therefore priority setting is likely to remain a key element of any enduring healthcare commissioning function.

Box 3.1: Features of priority setting/resource allocation in health and social care in England

Healthcare
- Revenue generated primarily through direct taxation
- Budgets set at the national level
- Few user charges at the point of delivery
- Population-level resource allocation decisions made by commissioners
- Transition from implicit to explicit rationing taking place
- Limited use of individual budgets

Social care
- Revenue generated through national and local taxation and means-tested co-payments
- Local government instrumental in budget setting and priority setting
- Resources constrained through assessment processes and eligibility criteria
- Direct payments and individual budgets prevalent

Ethical principles of priority setting

It is often claimed that services should be commissioned that are likely to be the most effective in meeting the needs of patients and service users. However, clarifying what we mean by this remains a challenge. Apart from dispute over the notion of 'need' (discussed in the previous chapter), those allocating public resources are also obliged to reflect considerations of fairness and distributional justice: in other words, to ensure that no one group or section of society receives more than their fair share at the expense of others. Therefore, we must also consider which needs are greatest and what minimum levels of provision everyone should be entitled to. More often than not, our stated or revealed priorities reflect a confusion of ethical principles. For example, the NHS was set up to embody the principle of egalitarianism, which holds that fairness and equity at a national level override all other considerations. However, this has begun to erode with the introduction of a more consumer-focused model of care in which the sovereign rights of the individual patient or service user take precedence over broader population-based considerations (Øvretveit, 1997). In the English NHS, the challenge of reconciling these two imperatives – both of which have intuitive validity – falls primarily with the priority-setting commissioner.

Accompanying this emphasis on the individual's rights and choices is a concomitant assertion of the individual's *responsibilities* in relation to well-being. This recalls the ethical concept of *desert*, which has become increasingly prevalent within the general healthcare lexicon (Dolan and Tsuzhiya, 2009). Put crudely, this approach holds that we should help most those who help themselves and, by implication, deprioritise those who take insufficient steps to ward off ill-health – for example through unhealthy lifestyle choices. Again, some may consider this reasonable in the context of scarce resources. However, given the unequal social distribution of disease and unhealthy lifestyles, such an approach is likely to exacerbate health inequalities. Here the commissioner must consider the competing imperative to reduce disparities in health profile resulting from the broader social determinants of health.

Advocates of evidence-based priority setting often extol the principle of *utilitarianism* (or utility maximisation) in resource allocation (Williams, 1998). From this perspective, the aim of commissioners should be to invest in areas that will generate the greatest improvements in overall health and quality of life. This approach is encapsulated in the guidance produced by the National Institute for Health and Clinical Excellence (NICE) in relation to new healthcare technologies. NICE adopts a utilitarian framework in as much as it advocates the principles of effectiveness and cost-effectiveness as the main measures of a treatment's value (Williams et al, 2007a). However, unless we are prepared to disregard considerations of fairness, individual choice and levels of need, it seems unlikely that a utilitarian stance can remove the requirement for ethical debate and trade-offs in resource allocation. Priority setters are therefore required to develop ethical frameworks that acknowledge and reflect the multiplicity of legitimate moral considerations at play. Box 3.2 gives a brief definition of the ethical concepts and perspectives typically evoked in relation to healthcare rationing. While these principles (and trade-offs between them) may previously have remained implicit and unacknowledged, the aspiration to explicit priority setting requires them to be more formally articulated and discussed by commissioners and stakeholders. Trade-offs between considerations of efficiency, justice and need are also a feature of social work but are more likely to be embedded in professional norms and practices as well as formal eligibility criteria (Bergmark, 1996).

Box 3.2: Ethical perspectives and principles in resource allocation

Communitarianism	The injunction to allocate resources according to collectively agreed citizen values.
Desert	The principle that individuals should be held responsible for their behaviour and that this should influence access to scarce resources.
Disease severity	The ethical principle that resources should be weighted towards those in greatest need or with the most severe conditions.
Efficiency	The concern to maximise outcomes from within a limited resource.
Egalitarianism	The ethical foregrounding of collective responsibility for fair distribution of resources.
Equity	The principle that equal people should be given equal treatment – and in some cases that those worse off should receive extra resources.
Fair innings	The ethical principle that resources should be distributed so as to distribute healthy years most evenly across a population.
Libertarianism	The ethical foregrounding of individual choice and reward, whereby patients are understood as consumers with rights and choices.
Rule of rescue	The imperative to save human life wherever possible.
Utilitarianism	The injunction to bring about the maximum level of utility (for example overall health gain).

Public involvement in priority setting

Given the absence of clarity over the ends of priority setting, it is often argued that extensive public involvement is required to resolve ethical disputes (Richardson, 2002). As well as helping to achieve much-needed clarity, engagement with citizens is also seen as a means of increasing democratic accountability and raising awareness of the difficulties faced by public sector decision makers operating with scarce resources (Litva et al, 2002; see also Chapter Nine, this volume). There are few if any recent prescriptions for effective priority setting that do not include public engagement, and yet in practice this remains rare in both healthcare and social care (Vergel and Ferguson, 2006; Menon et al, 2007; Sabik and Lie, 2008) and the evidence demonstrating public willingness to be involved remains mixed (Litva et al, 2002; Wiseman et al, 2003). This section considers methods and barriers for involving citizens in the allocation of scarce health and social care resources (and should be read in conjunction with Chapter Nine, this volume).

The terms 'involvement' and 'participation', as employed here, exclude passive models of public communication and consultation, instead focusing on approaches that engender meaningful dialogue between the public and decision makers (in this case commissioners) (Rowe and Frewer, 2005). Similarly, the terms 'public' and 'citizen' are preferred to 'patient', 'service user' or 'consumer' on the grounds that involvement in priority setting (the allocation of population resources by public bodies) is different from involvement of individuals in the purchasing and delivery of their own care (Lomas, 1997). There are a number of ways in which we might seek to elicit the values and preferences of citizens (Mullen and Spurgeon, 2000). Recent attention has focused on the need for deliberative approaches, as Abelson et al (2003, p 240) note:

> A common thread weaving through the current participation debate is the need for new approaches that emphasize two-way interaction between decision makers and the public as well as deliberation among participants. Increasingly complex decision making processes, it is argued, require a more informed citizenry that has weighed the evidence on the issue, discussed and debated potential decision options and arrived at a mutually agreed upon decision or at least one by which all parties can abide. An active, engaged citizen (rather than the passive recipient of information) is the prescription of the day.

Accordingly, the merits of deliberative public engagement mechanisms such as citizens' 'panels', 'juries', 'summits' and 'deliberative polling' have been discussed and assessed (Mitton et al, 2009). The key areas of commonality of these approaches are as follows:

• Each is applied in situations (such as healthcare rationing) where decisions are complex and contested, involving trade-offs and requiring public buy-in.
• Each places the need for informed deliberation at the heart of the engagement process. This invariably involves interactions in which knowledge is generated and developed and values and perceptions are challenged.
• Each (with the partial exception of deliberative polling) relies on repeat contact with relatively small numbers of participants.

However, there are a number of problems and difficulties associated with deliberative involvement in decision making. First, the evidence base on the various methods remains underdeveloped (Mitton et al, 2009). This means that decisions over their deployment are difficult to make. Second, deliberative exercises can be extremely costly and complex to both devise and implement and yet, because of the relatively small numbers involved, do not in themselves provide a democratic mandate for action. This is awkward territory for decision makers as involvement requires that decisions are open to being shaped by public preferences. Therefore, clear plans need to be in place to integrate such exercises with other decision inputs and engagement should be avoided when decisions are subject to strong government direction. Finally, it is important that deliberation is not employed as a means of coercion whereby genuine differences of perspective and principle are shoe-horned into an uncomfortable consensus for the convenience of the decision maker.

Overall, therefore, there are strong reasons for the involvement gap in priority setting, which relate to the difficulty, cost and risks associated with substantive engagement of the public in the complex and highly charged business of rationing. However, a number of factors point to the need for this gap to be addressed. Although there is a growing body of work that explores and assesses engagement methodologies, there remains little formal specification of the relative merits of these within the specific context of health and social care commissioning.

Evidence and decision analysis

In priority setting, the move to provide greater transparency and accountability in the decision-making process has led to a strong drive to increase the use of evidence-based practice. Evidence-based practice in priority setting tends to draw on a number of technocratic approaches, which rely on quantifiable epidemiologic, clinical and financial data to support decision making (Coast et al, 1996; Neumann, 2005). This section briefly introduces the range of decision analytic approaches to priority setting and critiques the 'evidence-based' model. A number of practical approaches are described, including economic evaluation, and programme budgeting and marginal analysis (PBMA). Finally, a map of existing information resources is provided (see Table 3.1).

Economic approaches

One of the key concepts in economics is that of opportunity cost. This represents the consequences foregone of choosing to allocate resources in one way rather than another. Economic analysis provides evidence on the costs and consequences of different alternatives and demonstrates which service would provide maximum benefit from the available resource. Thus, economics is concerned with the promotion of efficiency. Economic analysis can explore two types of efficiency, namely allocative and technical. Allocative efficiency is concerned with how budgets should be allocated to achieve greatest efficiency within a population. Technical efficiency is concerned with the efficient production of services (Drummond, 1991). Thus, the interest for allocative efficiency is in what services to provide, while for technical efficiency it is in providing services at the least possible cost. Economics offers two distinct approaches to commissioners to help them explore the efficiency of resource allocation decisions. These are economic evaluation and PBMA. The definitions of the key economic concepts discussed above are presented in Box 3.3.

Economic evaluation

Economic evaluation in health and social care is defined as 'the comparative analysis of alternative courses of action in terms of both their costs and consequences' (Drummond et al, 2005, p 9). There are three main types of economic evaluation: cost–effectiveness analysis (CEA), cost–utility analysis (CUA) and cost–benefit analysis (CBA). CEA and CUA are the most commonly used in health technology

Box 3.3: Key economic concepts

Opportunity cost: The value of the consequences forgone by choosing to deploy a resource in one way rather than its best alternative use – thus, it is what you do not choose that is the opportunity cost.

Benefit forgone = opportunity cost.
Goal is to minimise opportunity cost.

Allocative efficiency: Allocation of resources to maximise the level of population health (that is, situations in which either inputs or outputs are put to their best possible uses in the healthcare community). For example, interest is in how commissioners allocate expenditure across disease areas/patients to achieve maximum health gain. One question may be: what do we screen for?

Technical efficiency: Occurs when we produce the maximum possible sustained output for any given set of inputs. In the context of healthcare, the questions one may explore include: Are we providing a healthcare service at least possible cost to the NHS? Can we use nurse technicians instead of surgeons? What is the most efficient way to screen for breast cancer?

assessments (HTAs) to determine the cost–effectiveness of health and social care interventions (Drummond et al, 2005). One of the main strengths is that they consider both costs and consequences, and make direct comparisons with two or more interventions. Evaluations use an incremental approach, which explores the difference in costs and the difference in benefits (examples include life years saved or quality-adjusted life years [QALYs] gained – see Box 3.4 for brief definitions) of the interventions. A common approach used in economic evaluations is the Incremental Cost Effectiveness Ratio (ICER), which simply involves calculating the difference in cost by the difference in outcomes and reports the incremental cost required to obtain a given unit of benefit (that is, cost per QALY) (for a more detailed discussion, see Gold et al, 1996; Drummond et al, 2005). As mentioned above, economic evaluations are underpinned by the utilitarian principle of maximising health benefits.

The results obtained from economic evaluations are generally used in two ways: a 'league table' or a 'threshold' approach. The cost-effectiveness league table involves listing programmes in order of increasing ICER (Lord et al, 2004). Maximising health resources would involve allocating resources from the top of the table downwards until all available resources are exhausted. However, the ranking of ICERs is problematic as no direct comparison between services has been made and, as such, different approaches to evaluation are most likely to have occurred. Context-specific data are often required to make league tables useful to local priority setting processes. However, commissioners rarely have the resources or expertise to conduct local evaluations and, as such, rely on existing, less relevant, studies. There are very few examples of QALY league tables being

Box 3.4: Economic tools used to aid priority setting

Economic evaluation

This explores the cost and consequences of alternative treatments/services. Cost-effectiveness analysis (CEA) and cost-utility analysis (CUA) are the most widely used in technology assessment.

CEA addresses technical efficiency questions. It measures effectiveness in terms of natural effect or physical unit. Examples include: cost per lives saved; cost per complication avoided; cost per symptom-free day; cost per bed day saved.

CUA can address both technical and allocative efficiency questions. It measures effectiveness in terms of QALYs gained. Results are presented as cost per additional QALY gained.

Examples of economic evaluations that have used CEA and CUA can be found on both the HTA programme and the NICE websites (see www.hta.ac.uk and www.nice.org.uk respectively).

Programme budgeting and marginal analysis (PBMA)

PMBA is a framework that draws on evidence and stakeholder engagement to explore priority-setting decisions. Programme budgeting looks at how resources are currently allocated. Marginal analysis is used to assess costs and benefits of potential reallocation or changes to current funding.

Quality-adjusted life year (QALY)

A QALY is a composite measure of health benefit that combines data on both the quality (morbidity) and the length of life (mortality).

used in priority setting. The most familiar one is the Oregon experiment, which is famous for its failure rather than success, with the rankings it produced being considered clinically counterintuitive (Hadorn, 1991).

An alternative way to present results is by comparing the ICER to a 'critical threshold value'. The aim here is to maximise health benefits from available resources and, as such, this should represent the marginal opportunity cost of the available resources (or budget) (Lord et al, 2004). This approach is used by NICE, which has a threshold of around £30,000 cost per QALY (Raftery, 2001). Despite the growing interest and number of economic evaluations available through bodies such as NICE, HTA work only makes recommendations on a small proportion of technologies and tends to be limited to new emerging drugs and medical devices. As such, NICE has tended to play a fairly limited role in resource allocation decisions locally, with a dearth of economic evidence available for the majority of health and social care spending. This makes decisions on disinvestment and reallocation of funds even more complex, as it is difficult to make the case to disinvest in programmes if evidence is lacking on clinical and cost–effectiveness (Pearson and Littlejohns, 2007; Elshaug et al, 2008; Elshaug et al, 2009). Further, although the number of economic evaluations in health has increased over recent years, there is an imbalance between evaluations for interventions for health and those for social care, with development of economic evaluation being much less in the latter (Knapp, 1999; McDaid et al, 2003). The lack of economic evidence is due largely to the complexity of many social welfare interventions, including 'a high degree of user involvement, significant variability within the programme, complex long term conditions and multiagency involvement' (McDaid et al, 2003, p 96).

A major issue for local decision makers is the time and cost involved in undertaking evaluations that are often not feasible or relevant for all resource allocation questions (Donaldson and Mooney, 1991). Economic evaluations tend to take on the utilitarian concern with maximising health, with little concern for the range of other social values detailed earlier. Further, economic evaluations traditionally make little reference to affordability and, in practice, the additional health gains in the ICER often come with additional costs. If implementation of cost-effectiveness interventions continues without consideration of the affordability to the health and social care system, then within the constraints of limited resources, this will lead to an increase in spending and/or inefficient allocation of resources. Research into the use of economic evaluations also highlights a number of further cultural, institutional and political barriers to the adoption of methods by decision makers (Williams and Bryan, 2007; Eddama and Coast, 2009).

Programme budgeting and marginal analysis (PBMA)

PBMA is a framework put forward for priority setting and has been increasingly used in healthcare in the UK and internationally (Brambleby, 1995; Mitton et al, 2003; Mitton and Donaldson, 2004; Bate and Mitton, 2006; Donaldson et al, 2006). The Department of Health (DH) has advocated its use in commissioning and priority setting in recent years (DH, 2009). The DH also provides a free resource to local commissioners, which enables them to undertake programme budgeting on 23 different disease areas (DH, 2010). In short, programme budgeting allows for exploration of resource usage and analysis in relation to effectiveness and efficiency (Novick, 1965). Marginal analysis enables comparison of the costs and outputs of programmes (Mitton and Donaldson, 2003). The concept here is around assessing costs and benefits at 'the margin' and the focus is on 'benefit gained from the next unit of resources or lost from having one unit less' (Donaldson et al, 2010, p 2). Although there are a number of PBMA formats, the framework basically asks a series of five questions around resource usage (Donaldson et al, 2010, p 4):

1. What resources are available in total?
2. In what ways are these resources currently being spent?
3. What are the main candidates for more resources and what would be their effectiveness and cost?
4. Are there any areas of care within the programme that could be provided to the same level of effectiveness but with less resources, so releasing those resources to fund candidates from (3) (technical efficiency)?
5. Are there areas of care that, despite being effective, should have less resources because a proposal (or proposals) from (3) is (are) more effective for the resources spent (allocative efficiency)?

PBMA therefore involves the use of programme budgeting to identify areas for change in current practice. The framework also involves the establishment of an expert panel who draw on local knowledge and evidence to assess the impact of proposed changes (as per questions 3 to 5) (Mitton and Donaldson, 2003). Thus, a number of resources – including economic evaluations, needs assessments, reviews of local and national policy, health professionals, and patient and service user views – can be used to aid decision making and determine priorities (Cohen, 1994; Craig et al, 1995; Ruta et al, 1996).

PBMA is not without its critics and one of the problems associated with this approach relates to operational difficulties. PBMA is both time and resource intensive and there is often a lack of available good-quality data to inform the process (Donaldson and Mooney, 1991; Twaddle and Walker, 1995). While PBMA may provide a platform for engagement and allow for a sense of ownership over the decision-making process (Ruta et al, 2005), securing engagement from all relevant parties can be difficult (Mitton et al, 2003; Robinson et al, 2011). Some of the major barriers to PBMA relate to organisational culture. Lack of organisational stability, changes in personnel, restructuring of services and the absence of a culture receptive to change are all aspects that have limited the success of PBMA (Mitton et al, 2003). Furthermore, evidence suggests that even when stakeholders sign up to the PBMA approach, there are inherent difficulties in actually reallocating funds between very different programme areas, with a natural reluctance of providers to give up funds for investment in other areas (Twaddle and Walker, 1995; Robinson et al, 2011). Overall, technocratic processes and a strong evidence base are important elements of priority setting. However, the effective use of evidence, information and analysis depends on the range of other factors presented here, including: the information and analytical skill-set of decision makers; the presence of a receptive organisational and political climate for an evidence-based approach; and resolution of political and ethical conflicts.

Health and social care resources available to commissioning teams

There are a number of existing health and social care resources that provide information on different types of economic data. For example, the NICE and HTA programme websites (see www.nice.org.uk and www.hta.ac.uk respectively) provide details of economic evaluations of technologies that have been conducted nationally. Other sites such as the Health Economics Evaluations Database (HEED) contain details of both national and internationally published studies that have used economic methods and approaches. The DH provides tools and resources that allow commissioners to undertake local programme budgeting exercises. Table 3.1 provides more detail of the organisations and types of economic information available to commissioners.

Table 3.1: Existing health and social care resources available to commissioning teams (details on available resource are taken directly from organisations' websites)

Organisation	Outline of available resource	Website
National Institute for Health and Clinical Excellence (NICE)	Provides guidance on the clinical and cost-effectiveness of new and existing medicines, treatments and procedures in the NHS	www.nice.org.uk/
Social Care Institute for Excellence (SCIE), an independent charity, funded by the DH and the devolved administrations in Wales and Northern Ireland	Identifies and disseminates the knowledge base for good practice in social care	www.scie.org.uk/
Health Technology Assessment (HTA) programme	The HTA programme produces independent research about the effectiveness of different healthcare treatments and tests for those who use, manage and provide care in the NHS	www.hta.ac.uk/
Health Economic Evaluations Database (HEED)	Contains extensive information on national and international studies that have conducted economic evaluations of treatments and medical interventions	http://heed.wiley.com
Centre for Reviews and Dissemination (CRD), based at the University of York and part of the National Institute for Health Research	Undertakes systematic reviews that evaluate the effects of health and social care interventions It also is home to the following databases – DARE, HTA and NHS EED – which provide details on economic reviews and HTAs	www.york.ac.uk/inst/crd/
NHS Evidence	Provides extensive access to studies conducted in health and social care.	www.evidence.nhs.uk
NHS information available to NHS staff	Programme budgeting commissioning tools	www.dh.gov.uk/programmebudgeting NHSnet version – www.nchod.nhs.uk http://www.ic.nhs.uk/nhscomparators
The NHS Information Centre	Collects, analyses and presents national data and statistical information in health and social care	www.ic.nhs.uk/
NHS reference costs	NHS reference costs are published yearly and provide information on NHS expenditure, including unit costs, average length of stay and activity levels	www.dh.gov.uk
Personal Social Services Research Unit (PSSRU)	Provides data on the unit costs of health and social care, which can be used in economic evaluations	www.pssru.ac.uk/

Source: Details on available resources are taken directly from organisations' websites

Accountability for reasonableness

Given the multiplicity of available ethical principles to inform priority setting and the need to combine social values with other drivers of decisions, recent attention has turned to notions of procedural justice and the need for fair decision-making *processes*. Currently, the most prominent of these is 'Accountability for Reasonableness' (A4R) (Daniels and Sabin, 2008). A4R incorporates elements of *communitarianism* in its commitment to deliberation and commonly agreed value propositions in the allocation of scarce resources. The framework is made up of four conditions of fair process, which, if met in full, should obviate the requirement for a single guiding ethical principle. The key to A4R is the requirement to include publicity, deliberation and appeal (as well as information and evidence) in priority-setting processes. This approach considers a process as fair if it is able to demonstrate transparency, allows for revision and 'appeals to rationales that all can accept as relevant' (Daniels, 2000, p 1300). By following such a process it is proposed that unpopular decisions are more likely to be accepted by stakeholders.

Although authors have questioned the extent to which A4R resolves the problem of value pluralism (Friedman, 2008), it has proved useful to decision makers seeking to formalise their processes, including commissioners in England (Martin et al, 2002; Robinson et al, 2009). However, a weakness of the A4R framework is the limited degree of democratic legitimacy conferred by adherence to its conditions (Friedman, 2008; Kapiriri et al, 2009). Therefore, in order for commissioners to become trusted guardians of the public purse, more involvement and engagement is required as well as other strategies for increasing the legitimacy of the rationing enterprise (Williams et al, 2007b).

Politics and systems

In the discussion up to now we hope to have demonstrated the importance of ethics, involvement, evidence and process to priority setting in commissioning. However, we also hope to have raised sufficient doubts in relation to each of these to suggest that the 'solutions' to the rationing problem need to be sophisticated and multifaceted: the realities of pluralism, uncertainty and methodological failure demand that this is the case. However, even where commissioners have devised decision criteria and processes that they consider to be evidence based, inclusive and fair, more work is required if these are to be accepted and enacted in full. This section is concerned with two important factors affecting the success of priority setting: *legitimacy* and *implementation*. These are important because without legitimacy (that is, the general perception that rationing decisions are fair and reasonable) the most robust of decision-making processes will remain subject to attack, and unless they are *actually implemented*, priority-setting decisions and processes are effectively redundant.

The challenges facing rationers when seeking to implement policy decisions can be illustrated through application of Matland's (1995) ambiguity–conflict model (see Figure 3.1). According to Matland, approaches to implementation should reflect the extent of ambiguity and conflict surrounding a policy. Where these measures are both low (that is, there is clarity over aims and little or no disagreement between those involved), a rational, linear approach to implementation might reasonably be adopted. In these circumstances, implementation is characterised as 'administrative' and depends in most part on availability of resources. In conditions of low ambiguity and high conflict (that is, where the aims of policy are clear but disputed), the approach to implementation will require some exercise of either power or negotiation – for example through sanctions or incentives for compliance. In cases of low conflict and high ambiguity, policies are likely to be implemented in an experimental fashion, with emphasis, at least in the short term, on learning rather than results. Finally, policies marked by high ambiguity and high conflict are likely to be dependent on coalitions of actors at the local level for their implementation, with reduced scope for central control.

One might postulate that as rationing decisions involve removal or withholding of potentially beneficial interventions, they will invariably be surrounded by significant levels of conflict as those who 'lose out' (as patients, producers or professionals) will object. As we have seen, it is also typical for priority-setting activities to lack clarity of purpose – as multiple objectives, principles and influences are brought to bear on decisions. Rationing decisions frequently therefore fall into the category of high ambiguity and high conflict, and this goes some way towards explaining why the 'nettle' of explicit rationing is rarely grasped in full. Instead, compromises are sought and definitive statements of purpose are avoided in order to maintain a fragile peace between stakeholders at local and national levels. Indeed, NICE can be seen as an example of how attempts to reduce ambiguity (by adopting clear decision criteria) can increase conflict (Syrett, 2003).

So how is this manifest in practice? All too often, local commissioners are given insufficient clarity from political overseers with respect to the aims and criteria of rationing (Klein et al, 1996) and, as we have seen, this shortfall is not currently mitigated by public engagement. Without a clearer conception of aims, decisions (and their implementation) are more likely to be influenced by bargaining between local interest groups, making power an important consideration in both health and social care contexts (Blackman and Atkinson, 1997; Milewa

Figure 3.1: Matland's (1995) ambiguity-conflict model

	Low conflict	**High conflict**
Low ambiguity	Administrative implementation *Resources*	Political implementation *Power*
High ambiguity	Experimental implementation *Contextual conditions*	Symbolic implementation *Coalition strength*

Source: Matland (1995)

and Barry, 2005). Decision makers may also experience resistance and blockages from within frontline, implementing organisations – any priority-setting function or process will be located in a broader decision, delivery and performance management system and this context will therefore impact on the success or otherwise of its operations and outputs. Although there is a substantial literature on healthcare organisations and institutions, relatively little is known about the specific implications of these for local-level priority setting. As a result, much of the responsibility for designing local systems has been left to commissioners themselves. This leads potentially to significant variation in relation to factors such as: the remit and 'clout' of priority-setting bodies; the stated role and expectation of individual participants; and the linkage between determinations reached and actual resource allocation processes within and across organisations. The risk is that commissioners fail to securely embed priority setting within organisational (and interorganisational) systems (Williams and Bryan, 2007). Clearly, this is an area of crucial importance if priority setting is to become an integral component of commissioning (and joint commissioning) within the NHS.

The ambiguity and conflict surrounding priority setting also require those organising and supporting local processes to move beyond narrow conceptions of leadership associated with previous models of governance (O'Flynn, 2007). As well as being accountable upwardly to government and national policy bodies such as NICE, local leaders must also engage a plethora of local stakeholders and citizens, and 'manage the message' of priority setting in a difficult economic climate. Far from being a purely technical or procedural process, therefore, priority setting requires political acumen and skills in relationship management and coalition building so that 'tough choices' can be taken and implemented without undermining trust in healthcare institutions. The extent to which such leadership skills are evident will therefore be important in determining the success of any priority-setting endeavour. However, it is hard to escape the conclusion that a strong mandate is required from the centre – that is, government – if such difficult choices are to have legitimacy and are to be fully implemented and enforced at local levels.

Conclusions

Early sections of this chapter described the multiplicity of principles by which priority-setting decisions might be made and considered the overall ethics of priority setting. They also introduced a series of ethical principles and explained how these are currently invoked and applied in priority-setting debates and prescriptions. Commentators have noted the irreducible plurality in the ethics of priority setting and the need therefore for engagement with the public over values. However, mobilising the public as citizens with a stake in priority-setting decisions is both technically difficult and politically fraught. Genuinely 'shared' decisions require the public to be aware of the principles of scarcity and opportunity cost and to operate under the Rawlsian 'veil of ignorance' (Rawls,

1972) (that is, decision makers do not know their own personal circumstances – wealth, age, gender, education and so on – and as such make decisions through a 'veil of ignorance'). This is said to be fair as decision makers deliberate without personal bias, since they realise they could be *anybody* in a society. This implies the need for deliberative approaches in which trade-offs, ethical dilemmas and scarcity can be confronted and discussed. Despite the challenges posed by these requirements, the move to explicit decision making suggests that the legitimacy provided by public and stakeholder buy-in to decisions will become increasingly important for commissioners.

However, public involvement should sit alongside other decision influences – notably evidence and analysis – and this chapter has briefly introduced some of the key approaches to decision analysis while acknowledging the limitations of these. Much of the literature pertaining to healthcare priority setting is strongly influenced by the discipline of economics and focuses on the ways in which particular forms of economic evidence are used to inform and shape priority-setting processes. However, it is increasingly accepted that economic models, while instructive, are insufficient to meet the complex needs of health and social care priority setting in contemporary, developed-world health systems. The added value of decision models such as PBMA and A4R has also been discussed. In contrast to health, social care has remained largely absent from discussions of the priority-setting function (both generally and specifically in relation to commissioning). There is therefore less clarity in terms of what the role of priority setting in social care is and should be. Although the narrative of collective population-based decision making appears to have less purchase in social care settings, the resource gaps remain (at least) as severe, suggesting that this is an area that requires greater attention.

Overall, the current political and economic context has highlighted the need for explicit and fair priority setting, and in many countries commissioners have emerged as the primary decision-making agent in this process. It is important and timely, therefore, to develop a broad and in-depth understanding of current practices so that informed prescriptions for improvement can be formulated. However, conflict and ambiguity – in terms of ethics, processes, evidence, organisations, institutions and politics – dictate that any such prescriptions will need to take account of the contingency of priority setting on local context, and therefore the absence of a 'magic bullet' or 'one-size-fits-all' recipe for improvement.

Further reading

- Klein, R., Day, P. and Redmayne, S. (1996) *Managing scarcity: priority setting and rationing in the National Health Service*, Maidenhead: Open University Press – provides a good account of the theory and history of priority setting.
- McDaid, D., Byford, S. and Sefton, T. (2003) *Because it's worth it: a practical guide to conducting economic evaluations in the social welfare field*, York: Joseph Rowntree Foundation – offers a practical guide to conducting economic evaluations in the field of social welfare.
- Mitton, C. and Donaldson, C. (2004) *The priority setting toolkit: a guide to the use of economics in health care decision making*, London: BMJ – provides a practical guide to conducting PBMA in priority setting.
- Williams, I., Robinson, S. and Dickinson, H. (2011) *Rationing in health care: the theory and practice of priority setting*, Bristol: The Policy Press – brings together the theories and practice of priority setting and presents this in a way that is practical and accessible for students and professionals.

Useful websites

See Table 3.1 for a summary.

Reflective exercises

1. Having read this chapter, how should priority-setting decisions connect to actual resource allocation processes?
2. Think about a particular priority-setting process or rationing decision that you have been involved in or read about. What role should different types of evidence play in resource allocation decisions?
3. What ethical framework/s should inform priority setting?
4. What is (and perhaps should be) the role of citizens in establishing decision processes, criteria and outcomes?

References

Abelson, J. (2003) 'Deliberations about deliberative methods: issues in the design and evaluation of public participation processes', *Social Science and Medicine*, vol 57, no 2, pp 239-51.

Bate, A. and Mitton, C. (2006) 'Application of economic principles in healthcare priority setting', *Expert Review Pharmacoeconomics and Outcomes Research*, vol 6, no 3, pp 275-84.

Bergmark, A. (1996) 'Need, allocation and justice – on priorities in the social services', *Scandinavian Journal of Social Welfare*, vol 5, pp 45-56.

Blackman, T. and Atkinson, A. (1997) 'Needs targeting and resource allocation in community care', *Policy Studies*, vol 18, no 2, pp 125-38.

Brambleby, P. (1995) 'A survivor's guide to programme budgeting', *Health Policy*, vol 33, pp 127-45.

Cabinet Office (2010) *The coalition: our programme for government*, London: Cabinet Office, www.cabinetoffice.gov.uk/media/409088/pfg_coalition.pdf

Coast, J. (1997) 'The rationing debate: rationing within the NHS should be explicit: the case against', *British Medical Journal*, vol 314, pp 1114-18.

Coast, J. (2004) 'Is economic evaluation in touch with society's health values?', *British Medical Journal*, vol 329, pp 1233-6.

Coast, J., Donovan, J. L. and Frankel, S. J. (1996) *Priority setting: the health care debate*, Chichester: John Wiley & Sons.

Cohen, D. (1994) 'Marginal analysis in practice: an alternative to needs assessment health care', *British Medical Journal*, vol 309, pp 781-4.

Craig, N., Parkin, D. and Gerard, K. (1995) 'Clearing the fog on the Tyne: programme budgeting in Newcastle and North Tyneside Health Authority', *Health Policy*, vol 33, pp 107-25.

Daniels, N. (2000) 'Accountability for reasonableness: establishing a fair process for priority setting is easier than agreeing on principles', *British Medical Journal*, vol 321, pp 1300-1.

Daniels, N. and Sabin, J. (2008) *Setting limits fairly: learning to share resources for health*, Oxford: Oxford University Press.

DH (Department of Health) (2008) *Achieving the competencies: practical tips for NHS commissioners*, London: DH.

DH (2009) *World class commissioning handbook*, available online via www.dh.gov.uk/

DH (2010) *Programme budgeting commissioning tools*, available online via www. dh.gov.uk/programmebudgeting

Dolan, P. and Tsuzhiya, A. (2009) 'The social welfare function and individual responsibility: some theoretical issues and empirical evidence', *Journal of Health Economics*, vol 28, pp 210-20.

Donaldson, C. and Mooney, G. (1991) 'Needs assessment, priority setting, and contracts for health care: an economic view', *British Medical Journal*, vol 303, pp 1529-30.

Donaldson, C., Bate, A., Mitton, C., Peacock, S., Ruta, D. (2006) 'Priority setting in the public sector: turning economics into a management process', in J. Hartley (ed) *Managing improvement in public service delivery: progress and challenges*, Cambridge: Cambridge University Press.

Donaldson, C., Bate, A., Mitton, C., Dionne, F. and Ruta, D. (2010) 'Rational disinvestment', *QJM*, vol 103, no 10, pp 801-7.

Drummond, M. (1991) 'Output measurement for resource-allocation decisions in health care', in A. McGuire, P. Fenn and K. Mayhew (eds) *Providing health care: the economics of alternative systems of finance and delivery*, Oxford: Oxford University Press.

Drummond, M. F., Sculpher, M. J., Torrance, G. W., O'Brien, B. J. and Stoddart, G. L. (2005) *Methods for the economic evaluation of health care programmes*, Oxford: Oxford University Press.

Eddama, O. and Coast, J. (2009) 'Use of economic evaluation in local health care decision-making in England: a qualitative investigation', *Health Policy*, vol 89, no 3, pp 261-70.

Elshaug, A. G., Hiller, J. E. and Moss, J. R. (2008) 'Exploring policymakers' perspectives on disinvestment from ineffective health care practices', *International Journal of Technology Assessment in Health Care*, vol 24, no 1, pp 1-9.

Elshaug, A.G., Moss, J. R., Littlejohns, P., Karnon, J., Merlin, T. L. and Hiller, J. E. (2009) 'Identifying existing health care services that do not provide value for money', *Medical Journal of Australia*, vol 190, pp 269-73.

Friedman, A. (2008) 'Beyond accountability for reasonableness', *Bioethics*, vol 22, no 2, pp 101-12.

Gold, M. R., Siegel, J. E., Russell, L. B. and Weinstein, M. C. (eds) (1996) *Cost-effectiveness in health and medicine*, New York, NY: Oxford University Press.

Hadorn, D. C. (1991) 'Setting health priorities in Oregon: cost-effectiveness meets the rule of rescue', *Journal of the American Medical Association*, vol 265, pp 2218-25.

Kapiriri, L., Norheim, O. F. and Martin, D. K. (2009) 'Fairness and accountability for reasonableness: do the views of priority setting decision makers differ across health systems?', *Social Science and Medicine*, vol 68, pp 766-73.

Klein, R., Day, P. and Redmayne, S. (1996) *Managing scarcity: priority setting and rationing in the National Health Service*, Maidenhead: Open University Press.

Knapp, M. (1999) 'Economic evaluation and mental health: sparse past ... fertile future?', *Journal of Mental Health Policy and Economics*, vol 2, no 4, pp 163-7.

Litva, A., Coast, J., Donovan, J., Eyles, J., Shepherd, M., Tacchi, J., Abelson, J. and Morgan, L. (2002) 'The public is too subjective: public involvement at different levels of health-care decision making', *Social Science and Medicine*, vol 54, pp 1825–37.

Lomas, J. (1997) 'Reluctant rationers: public input into health care priorities', *Journal of Health Services Research and Policy*, vol 2, pp 103-11.

Lord, J., Laking, G. and Fischer, A. (2004) 'Health care resource allocation: is the threshold rule good enough?', *Journal of Health Services Research and Policy*, vol 9, no 4, pp 237-45.

Martin, D. K., Giacomini, M. and Singer, P. A. (2002) 'Fairness, accountability for reasonableness, and the views of priority setting decision-makers', *Health Policy*, vol 61, pp 279-90.

Matland, R. E. (1995) 'Synthesising the implementation literature: the ambiguity-conflict model of policy implementation', *Journal of Public Administration Research and Theory*, vol 5, no 2, pp 145-57.

McDaid, D., Byford, S. and Sefton, T. (2003) *Because it's worth it: a practical guide to conducting economic evaluations in the social welfare field*, York: Joseph Rowntree Foundation.

Mechanic, D. (1995) 'Dilemmas in rationing health care services: the case for implicit rationing', *British Medical Journal*, vol 310, pp 1655-9.

Menon, D., Stafinski, T. and Martin, D. (2007) 'Priority-setting for healthcare: who, how and is it fair?', *Health Policy*, vol 84, pp 220-33.

Milewa, T. and Barry, C. (2005) 'Health policy and the politics of evidence', *Social Policy and Administration*, vol 39, no 5, pp 498-512.

Mitton, C. and Donaldson, C. (2003) 'Tools of the trade: a comparative analysis of approaches to priority setting in healthcare', *Health Services Management Research*, vol 16, pp 96-105.

Mitton, C. and Donaldson, C. (2004) 'Health care priority setting: principles, practice and challenges', *Cost Effectiveness and Resource Allocation*, vol 2, no 3, doi:10.1186/1478-7547-2-3.

Mitton, C., Peacock, S., Donaldson, C. and Bate, A. (2003) 'Using PBMA in health care priority setting: description, challenges and experience', *Applied Health Economics and Health Policy*, vol 2, no 3, pp 121-34.

Mitton, C., Smith, N., Peacock, S., Evoy, B. and Abelson, J. (2009) 'Public participation in health care priority setting: a scoping review', *Health Policy*, vol 91, no 3, pp 219-28.

Mooney, G. (1998) '"Communitarian claims" as an ethical basis for allocating health care resources', *Social Science and Medicine*, vol 4, no 9, pp 1171-80.

Mullen, P. and Spurgeon, P. (2000) *Priority setting and the public*, Oxford: Radcliffe Medical Press.

Neumann, P. (2005) *Using cost effectiveness analysis to improve health care: opportunities and barriers*, New York, NY: Oxford University Press.

Newdick, C. (2005) *Who should we treat? Rights, rationing and resources in the NHS* (2nd edition), Oxford: Oxford University Press.

Novik, D. (1965) *Program budgeting: program analysis and the federal budget*, Cambridge, MA: Harvard University Press.

O'Flynn, J. (2007) 'From New Public Management to public value: paradigmatic change and managerial implications', *Australian Journal of Public Administration*, vol 66, no 3, pp 353-66.

Øvretveit, J.A. (1997) 'Managing the gap between demand and publicly affordable health care in an ethical way', *European Journal of Public Health*, vol 7, no 2, pp 128-35.

Pearson, S. and Littlejohns, P. (2007) 'Reallocating resources: how should the National Institute for Health and Clinical Excellence guide disinvestment efforts in the National Health Service?', *Journal of Health Services Research and Policy*, vol 12, pp 160-5.

Raftery, J. (2001) 'NICE: faster access to modern treatments? Analysis of guidance on health technologies', *British Medical Journal*, vol 323, pp 1300-3.

Rawls, J. (1972) *A theory of justice*, Oxford: Oxford University Press.

Richardson, J. (2002) 'The poverty of ethical analysis in economics and the unwarranted disregard of evidence', in C. Murray and A. Lopez (eds) *Summary measures of population health*, Geneva: World Health Organization, pp 627-40.

Robinson, S., Dickinson, H. and Williams, I. (2009) *Evaluation of the prioritisation process at South Staffordshire PCT*, Birmingham: Health Services Management Centre.

Robinson, S., Dickinson, H., Williams, I., Freeman, T., Rumbold, B. and Spence, K. (2011) *Setting priorities in health: A study of English Primary Care Trusts*, London: Nuffield Trust.

Rowe, G. and Frewer, L. J. (2005) 'A typology of public engagement mechanisms', *Science, Technology and Human Values*, vol 30, p 251.

Russell, J. and Greenhalgh, T. (2009) *Rhetoric, evidence and policy making: a case study of priority setting in primary care*, London: UCL.

Ruta, D. A., Donaldson, C. and Gilray, I. (1996) 'Economics, public health and health care purchasing: the Tayside experience', *Journal of Health Services Research and Policy*, vol 1, no 4, pp 185-93.

Ruta, D.A., Mitton, C., Bate, A. and Donaldson, C. (2005) 'Programme budgeting and marginal analysis: bridging the divide between doctors and managers', *British Medical Journal*, vol 330, pp 1501-3.

Sabik, L. M. and Lie, R. K. (2008) 'Priority setting in health care: lessons from the experiences of eight countries', *International Journal for Equity and Health*, vol 7, no 4, doi:10.1186/1475-9276-7-4.

Scourfield, P. (2007) 'Social care and the modern citizen: client, consumer, service user, manager and entrepreneur', *British Journal of Social Work*, vol 37, pp 107-22.

Syrett, K. (2003) 'A technocratic fix to the "legitimacy problem"? The Blair government and health care rationing in the United Kingdom', *Journal of Health Politics, Policy and Law*, vol 28, no 4, pp 715-46.

Twaddle, S. and Walker, A. (1995) 'Programme budgeting and marginal analysis: application within programmes to assist purchasing in Greater Glasgow Health Board', *Health Policy*, vol 33, pp 91-105.

Vergel, Y. B. and Ferguson, B. (2006) 'Difficult commissioning choices: lessons from English primary care trusts', *Journal of Health Services Research and Policy*, vol 11, no 3, pp 150-4.

Williams, A. (1998) 'Economics, QALYs and medical ethics: a health economist's perspective', in S. Dracopoulou (ed) *Ethics and values in health care management*, London: Routledge.

Williams, I. and Bryan, S. (2007) 'Cost-effectiveness analysis and formulary decision making in England: findings from research', *Social Science and Medicine*, vol 65, pp 2116-29.

Williams, I., Bryan, S. and McIver, S. (2007a) 'Health technology coverage decisions: evidence from the N.I.C.E. "experiment" in the use of cost-effectiveness analysis', *Journal of Health Services Research and Policy*, vol 12, no 2, pp 73-79.

Williams, I., Durose, J., Peck, E., Dickinson, H. and Wade, E. (2007b) *How can PCTs shape, reflect and increase public value?*, Birmingham: Health Services Management Centre.

Williams, I., Robinson, S. and Dickinson, H. (2011) *Rationing in health care: the theory and practice of priority setting*, Bristol: The Policy Press.

Wiseman, V., Mooney, G., Berry, G., and Tang, K. C. (2003) 'Involving the general public in priority setting: experiences from Australia', *Social Science and Medicine*, vol 56, pp 1001-12.

FOUR

Procurement and market management

Chris Lonsdale

Summary

This chapter explores:
- key elements of the procurement process;
- how organisations decide what they need and select/manage suppliers;
- issues of trust, opportunism and power;
- key lessons for future procurement practice.

While the coalition government has stated its intention to implement radical change within the United Kingdom (UK) health and social care sectors (DH, 2010), in particular, by abolishing NHS primary care trusts (PCTs) and replacing them with general practitioner (GP) consortia, some principles will continue to form the basis of any commissioner's expertise. The commercial principles related to procurement are examples of these and are the subject of this chapter. Its aim is to provide an overview of the core principles and consider their implications for practice, making reference in the process to the practical challenges of health and social care commissioning. In doing so, the chapter also aims to rectify the tendency within the health and social care literature for debate over procurement policy and practice to exist in isolation from the concepts and frameworks within the broader procurement and associated literature.

A question often asked by public sector managers concerns the difference between commissioning and procurement. The answer very much depends on the definitions given to the two terms. It is not the intention here to discuss what those different definitions might be (see the Introduction to this volume for further detail). However, it is worth pointing out that in the procurement and supply management literature, the procurement process is commonly thought to include decisions related to the internal assessment of need and the development of product or service specifications (Hughes et al, 1998; Lonsdale and Watson, 2005). The view taken is that such decisions are often critical to the ultimate success of a procurement exercise and that procurement managers should, as a result, very much see involvement in such decisions as a core part of their remit.

If this steer from the procurement literature is accepted, a high-level version of the procurement process can be mapped out thus:

- the identification of need;
- the development of a specification (input, output or outcome based);
- a market search, for suitable bidders;
- the running of a competitive process, sometimes involving negotiation;
- provider selection;
- the development of a contract (more or less formal);
- the monitoring and improvement of supplier performance.

If the purchase is a repeat purchase, then a number of these steps might be omitted, particularly in the private sector where the buying organisation may decide to extend the relationship without running another competition (Robinson et al, 1967).

The aim of this process is, of course, best value for money (VFM). Best VFM is not understood as the lowest price bid (although that is what many organisations often opt for), but as the achievement of the required functionality for the lowest possible (and advisable) whole life cost (Cox, 2005). While the economic concept of 'surplus value' (the gap between the supplier's costs of production and the buyer's valuation of a product or service) is not easily transferred to the organisational buying arena, it can be said that if a buying organisation has indeed been successful in achieving best VFM, it has obtained most of the surplus value as consumer surplus. This is true whether the relationship is relatively 'arm's-length' or one that is more collaborative. The difference in the latter case is that collaboration between the buyer and the supplier increases the amount of surplus value to be divided in the transaction.

The question then arises over what principles and practices will allow buying organisations, or, in the present context, commissioning organisations, to obtain best VFM. While it is a rather crude divide, this chapter answers this question in two parts. First, reflecting the aforementioned steer from the procurement literature, the author considers some of the internal challenges to obtaining best VFM. Having explored these, the author then proceeds to the challenges of supplier selection and management.

The challenge of internal management

The first steps of the procurement process concern the assessment of need (see also Chapter Two, this volume) and the development of a specification (which can, in turn, also imply a supplier preference). Both of these tasks, part of what is referred to in the procurement literature as 'internal demand management' (Lonsdale and Watson, 2005), are central to the success of any procurement exercise as they will affect the nature and quantity of demand and the ease with which the buying organisation will be able to negotiate and contract with suppliers for that demand (that is, the procurement understanding of the term 'demand management' is not dissimilar from that in the health and social care literature). However, internal demand management is not straightforward and often done badly by buying organisations in both the public and the private sectors (Russill, 2003; Smith, 2003; Ellinor, 2007; Gilbert, 2007). In order to understand why this might be the case, we need to briefly access the organisational management literature.

Models of organisation

A prominent debate within this (and the wider management) literature concerns the extent to which organisations operate in a rational manner. In a rational organisation, all necessary information is collected, senior managers analyse it and then come to decisions that reflect the analysis. These decisions are then accepted by employees who are dedicated to assisting their organisation to achieve its agreed-upon objectives. In sum, organisational objectives, cause and effect are unambiguous and employees orderly. Not surprisingly, much of the organisational management literature finds this picture unconvincing. As a result, an alternative perspective, summarised by Pfeffer (1981) as a 'political model', has become popular.

The political model of organisations is largely the reverse of the rational model. First, it holds that, contrary to the claims of the rational model, information within organisations is often incomplete, for reasons of cost, inefficiency or strategic game playing. Second, and partly because of incomplete information, but also partly because of differing interests, it holds that there are often divisions among employees (including senior managers) regarding what the objectives of the organisation should be and how to achieve them. Third, in the model, conflict and bargaining among employees are common and expected, if not universally seen as legitimate. Finally, the outcomes of conflict and bargaining are said to be heavily influenced by organisational power. Relating this to decision making, the political model holds that organisations make decisions on the basis of incomplete information and that employees will often possess different interests and priorities (sometimes not in the overall interests of the organisation) and that they will often be willing to pursue them in a decision context mobilising their organisational power resources. All of these characteristics are said to affect the efficiency and effectiveness of organisations.

In terms of what causes different interests and priorities, the literature cites three factors in particular. The first is bounded rationality and relates back to the condition of incomplete information (Simon, 1957). It is argued that some employees innocently promote interests and priorities that clash with those of others and, more significantly, those of the organisation as a whole, as they are unable to appreciate the whole range of adverse consequences that will flow from them. They simply have limited information at their disposal and/or a limited capacity to analyse information and make informed judgements (March, 1994).

However, internal disagreements are not said to be due simply to bounded rationality and incomplete information. A second factor is said to be professional and functional cultures. It is argued that actors become socialised by their professional or functional role and that their interests and priorities are influenced by the values promoted by it (Freidson, 1986). It is said that such socialisation is not surprising given that employees gain qualifications, attend events, read publications and join associations and institutes all related to their profession or function. Such socialisation is said to be strong in the health and social care sectors (Mannion et al, 2005).

Finally, a third cause is cited – the principal-agent problem and self-interest. That is, the political model of organisations accepts the notion that some employees, on some occasions, will promote interests and priorities that they know to be detrimental to the overall welfare of their organisation in order to achieve their own personal or functional objectives (Pettigrew, 1977). This is often referred to within organisations as 'turf protection'. Public choice theorists, a tradition that applies economic models to public management and administration, have made a point of arguing that such behaviour is just as likely in the public sector as it is in the private sector (Hay, 2007).

Turning our attention to organisational power, said to be necessary for interests and priorities to be reflected in eventual decisions, three sources of power in particular emerge from the literature. These are hierarchical authority, centrality to the organisation's objectives (Hickson et al, 1971), sometimes referred to as 'horizontal' power resources (and based on the ideas of Emerson, 1962; see later in this chapter), and expertise (French and Raven, 1959). The idea is that, while in rational organisations common purpose and perfect information will lead to optimal decision making, in political organisations decision-making outcomes will often reflect the successful deployment of power resources and can, on occasions, have very little to do with the merits of the case (Pfeffer, 1981).

Therefore, the political model outlines two key and overlapping characteristics of organisations: incomplete information and conflicting interests and priorities. Incomplete information can prevent effective internal demand management for obvious reasons. It can cause managers to misjudge needs (not least by continuing to procure goods and services for which there is no longer a compelling requirement) and to fail to effectively specify goods and services (see Box 4.1 for a practical case study). Conflicting interests and priorities can also prevent effective internal demand management. A number of common problems caused by such conflicts have been identified, including the fragmentation of demand over an unnecessarily large number of suppliers, the over-specification of goods and services (often referred to as 'gold plating') and 'maverick' buying, the practice of using, usually favoured, suppliers that are not on an approved list (Lonsdale and Watson, 2005).

These problems can, in turn, lead to a number of different economic consequences (Lonsdale and Watson, 2005). First, organisations can suffer increased transaction costs, for example, if they use an unnecessarily large number of suppliers. Second, again if they employ a large number of suppliers, they can experience a loss of negotiation power, which, of course, can cause poor VFM.

> ## Box 4.1: Case example: information and mental health commissioning
>
> An example of how poor information is affecting NHS commissioning is provided in the area of mental health services. In a recent House of Commons Health Committee (2010) report into commissioning, the Royal College of Psychiatrists commented:
>
> > Local populations vary considerably in their mental health needs and commissioning should respond to that. But there is a lack of good quality local information on population needs, including unmet needs, which is important because those who are in most need may be less able to seek help. Poor use of evidence by commissioners may be the reason why the fivefold variation per person in the NHS budget for mental health services does not seem to follow known patterns of prevalence or need but appears to be almost random.
>
> *Source:* House of Commons Health Committee (2010, p 30)

Third, over-specification can lead to higher than necessary prices, something that can also be caused by maverick buying. Finally, organisations can miss opportunities to create innovative collaborative relationships, should demand be fragmented across an unnecessary number of suppliers.

Both of these characteristics, incomplete information and conflicts of interests and priorities, can be recognised within the UK healthcare commissioning environment. First, one of the main criticisms that has been levelled at the soon-to-be abolished PCTs is that they have often made commissioning decisions on a very poor information base and with very limited analytical skills. For example, the Care Quality Commission commented in 2010: 'In our work we have commonly identified significant concerns about the availability and use of relevant and reliable data to inform accurate assessments of service need' (House of Commons Health Committee, 2010, p 29). The House of Commons Health Committee (2010, p 29) report was also critical: 'It seems that many people in PCTs have no idea of how to use data. PCTs employ large numbers of staff, but too few of them seem to be able to analyse data effectively.' PCTs have also been criticised for often not providing GP practice-based commissioners with adequate or timely information (Cross, 2010).

It is clear that NHS commissioning has also been affected by conflicting interests and priorities. A number of examples can be given. First, there is evidence of both PCTs and GPs having 'favoured' providers (Brereton and Vasoodaven, 2010), something that it is said has led to PCTs not fully utilising their purchasing power. Second, some GPs have been said to be very resistant to take responsibility for demand management (Lewis and Dixon, 2005). Third, PCTs have been accused of inappropriately under-prioritising specialist care services (House of Commons Health Committee, 2010). Fourth, there has been inherent tension from GPs being both contributors to the management of, and suppliers to, PCTs.

Fifth, there is evidence of game playing, information withholding and sectional infighting within PCTs (Burnes and Pope, 2007). Sixth, there has been much disagreement concerning the provider functions of PCTs (House of Commons Health Committee, 2005). Finally, many local stakeholders have felt excluded from meaningful involvement in the commissioning process, with one mental health group quoted as saying: 'We are invited to attend [commissioning] meetings that discuss strategies. But our input is often overruled or ignored, and we are merely a box ticked' (Brereton and Vasoodaven, 2010, p 30).

This list does not paint a particularly happy picture of NHS commissioning. However, it is important to repeat the point made earlier that internal demand management problems are common in both the public and the private sectors. Indeed, evidence of information problems experienced elsewhere in the UK public sector is discussed below.

Managerial responses

In terms of addressing these shortcomings, a number of responses have been suggested. First, in terms of improved commissioning information and analytical skills, a number of recommendations have been made by experts in the field. These have included increased numbers of commissioners, higher remuneration for commissioners, in order to increase the numbers of high-quality staff, better use of information systems and the development of a culture that encourages staffing stability, so that commissioners can build up specialist expertise (House of Commons Health Committee, 2010). Of course, the coalition government's solution is to abolish PCTs and create more clinically dominated organisations (DH, 2010).

There is a broader comment to be made, however. The information and skills problem being faced by NHS commissioning organisations is only one of a number of similar problems being experienced right across the UK public sector. Numerous audit reports (for example, PAC, 2003, 2007; NAO, 2009) have pointed to situations where a policy that requires the UK public sector to act as an effective purchaser has been undermined by the UK government greatly underestimating, in terms of both staff numbers and experience, the task of creating an effective purchaser. As a result, it could be argued that governments can restructure areas of the public sector as many times as they like, but if none of the changes remedy the existence of an under-resourced and under-powered purchasing function, such changes are unlikely to be successful.

Second, the task of resolving internal conflicts is arguably even more intractable, as it often requires organisations to cease being political. As a result, recommendations might be better focused on coping within political organisations rather than seeking to transform them. In that spirit, it is perhaps most interesting to reflect on the options of those who lack hierarchical authority within an organisation. This, historically, has been the position of the procurement profession within most organisations (Smith, 2003). For those managing without hierarchical power, a number of principles are particularly important. The first is prioritisation. Particularly if a new procurement team has entered an organisation, there will be value in assessing whether 'quick wins' can be made in relatively uncontroversial areas of expenditure. Such wins could provide the team with credibility, something that will be an important attribute when more contentious areas of expenditure are tackled (Ellinor, 2007).

Second, an understanding of the drivers of conflicting interests and priorities can also provide value. In particular, it can alert a procurement team to the possibility that some conflicts are born of limited understanding, attention or information, contributing to bounded rationality, and can be resolved through engagement and discussion (Lonsdale and Watson, 2005). Of course, engagement and discussion will not usually, on their own, deliver results where a conflict is driven by the principal–agent problem. Here, alternative responses will be required. One such response might be alliance building (Lonsdale and Watson, 2005). Where a manager or department does not itself have internal power resources, it can 'borrow' those of others that are sympathetic to their perspective in the hope that their support will be reflected in the eventual decision. There can, therefore, be value in assessing which other managers or departments within the organisation have both a common mind and a degree of organisational influence. Alternatively, managers can decide not to seek to overcome conflicting interests and priorities, but, rather, seek a 'coalition of the willing' (Lonsdale and Watson, 2005). This can be a sensible course of action as evidence suggests that, for example, collaborative procurement projects can suffer from having too many participants (Moffatt, 2010). Again, this will require managers to undertake careful organisational analysis.

The challenge of supplier selection and management

The challenge of supplier selection and management is no less formidable than that faced internally within buying organisations. Some elements of this challenge are what might be referred to as technical. First, there is a need for a data template that allows for the systematic comparison of the commercial and clinical capabilities of shortlisted suppliers (Smith, 2009). Second, if an organisation is within a public or regulated sector, a thorough understanding of the European Union (EU) procurement rules is necessary. Third, a process that guides the performance management of suppliers and permits knowledge management is also required (Hughes, 2005). However, beyond these largely technical considerations, there are, as was the case with internal management, broad behavioural questions that managers within buying organisations must consider and, crucially, take a view on. The first of these concerns the concept of 'trust'. This is not with respect to the capabilities of the supplier, something referred to as 'competence trust'. It is rather the question of whether the buying organisation can trust the motivations of the supplier, something referred to as 'intentional trust' (Nooteboom, 2002). Again, the literature can assist our understanding.

Intentional trust, opportunism and procurement

The concept of 'intentional trust' is understood as the willingness of an actor to make itself vulnerable to the actions of another party, based on the expectation that the other party will behave honourably, irrespective of whether it is being monitored or otherwise controlled (Mayer et al, 1995). The advantages of intentional trust for procurement and supply management are many. It can lower transaction costs for both parties, including search costs, negotiating costs, contracting costs and monitoring costs. Through the willing exchange of product, service and process information, it can reduce the chance of the supplier not meeting the needs of the buying organisation (Chiles and McMakin, 1996). Finally, it can also eliminate the opportunity cost of the two parties not working closely together to increase the surplus value in the relationship. Effective collaboration has been shown to significantly increase innovation and problem solving in relationships and, as a result, enhance goods and services, reduce the cost of their delivery, or both (Webb and Hughes, 2009).

This is not to say that intentional trust can be developed straight away – something that can be a challenge for large-scale outsourcing projects, as such trust is needed immediately. Rather, it tends to be an outcome of a period of time when the buyer and supplier establish a track record of delivering on promises and acting in a cooperative manner (Hawkins, 2010). However, even when a supplier seems to be behaving in a manner whereby it is disinterested in exploiting buyer vulnerability, things may not always be what they appear. In short, a supplier may have opportunistic intentions and eventually these can show themselves (Williamson, 1985).

'Opportunism' has been defined as behaviour aimed at furthering self-interest and can be either blatant or subtle in nature (Williamson, 1996). 'Blatant opportunism' is understood as breaking (written or unwritten) contracts, lying, cheating or stealing. 'Subtle opportunism' is understood as self-interest seeking with guile and refers to acts whereby there is an incomplete or distorted disclosure of information, the aim of which is to mislead, confuse or disguise true intent. These two types of opportunism can either be on a large scale or represent efforts to 'tilt the system at the margins' and should be differentiated from 'simple self-interest seeking', whereby a supplier pursues its self-interest in a transparent manner (Williamson, 1985).

Examples of subtle opportunism include:

- adverse selection (whereby a supplier presents itself as a provider of goods or services of a quality that it has no intention of, or ability to, deliver);
- strategic misrepresentation (for example bluffing in negotiation);
- the promotion of asymmetrical lock-in (whereby a supplier deliberately engineers, and then exploits, a commercial arrangement whereby the buying organisation faces high barriers to exit from the relationship); and

- moral hazard (whereby a supplier either shirks or lowers quality in a manner that is not visible to the buying organisation).

All of these are seen as commonplace hazards in buyer–supplier relationships (Milgrom and Roberts, 1992).

If a buying organisation seeks to prevent or manage these types of opportunism then it is likely to incur high levels of transaction costs (that is, it will have to take great care during search and negotiation, afford itself considerable contractual protection and put considerable resources into providing monitoring; Chiles and McMakin, 1996). If it does not exercise such caution in the face of likely opportunism, it is likely to suffer instead considerable exploitation in the form of lower service or quality levels and/or higher prices (Milgrom and Roberts, 1992). A fear of opportunism can also hinder relationship development as both parties will be wary about entering into collaborative initiatives.

Buyer–supplier power relations and procurement

The second supplier-related behavioural issue concerns the impact of buyer–supplier power relations (Cox et al, 2000; see also Box 4.2 for a practical example). Do such power relations matter? Will suppliers exploit situations where the buying organisation is in a weak power position? The explicit message of various NHS reforms over the past 20 years suggests that buyer–supplier power relations do matter and that suppliers will exploit dominance where it is possessed. Indeed, key influences on health and social care policy over the past two decades, Bartlett and Le Grand, have been quoted as saying: 'A single dominant provider can

---

Box 4.2: Case example: the impact of commissioner–provider power

There is widespread acceptance that power affects the outcomes of commissioner–provider relationships. In the procurement of acute care in particular, this has caused problems for PCTs. For example, the House of Commons Select Committee (2010, p 35) recently commented:

[PCTs] struggle to make an impact as commissioners since there is a seemingly perennial imbalance of power between providers and commissioners. When the purchaser/provider split was introduced it was intended that purchasers would have the power that customers are supposed to have in real markets, where 'the customer is king.' However, it is often argued that, in practice, power has mainly resided with NHS providers. Dr David Colin-Thomé, the National Clinical Director for Primary Care at the [Department of Health], agreed that providers had retained a 'dominant position' and admitted that 'maybe we have made it worse' by being 'obsessed by the provider side' in policy development.

Source: House of Commons Health Committee (2010)

---

use its monopoly power to raise prices and to lower the quantity and quality of the services provided. Without the threat of competition it can afford to be unresponsive to the needs and wants of its consumers' (Bartlett and Le Grand, 1993, p 20). As a result, it is not surprising that commissioning organisations across the public sector have, over the past 20 years, been advised, for example, through an increased use of the 'third sector' and the greater adoption of internet-based procurement technology, to increase competition in their markets or, to use the favoured phrase, 'stimulate the market' (Gershon, 2004; DH, 2007; DCLG, 2008; Ernst & Young, 2009).

However, buyer–supplier power is not all about stimulating competition. This is because 'buyer–supplier power' is a relative concept. Power here is defined as the ability of one actor to make another actor behave in a manner it would not have otherwise done (Lukes, 1974). This ability, in turn, arises out of the relative possession of power resources. For Emerson (1962), the key power resources are utility (how important the transaction is to the two parties) and scarcity (what options outside of the transaction the two parties possess). Depending on the combination of resources held by the two parties, the power relations in the transaction can be supplier dominance, buyer dominance, independence or interdependence (Cox et al, 2000).

Those who claim that buyer–supplier power relations affect commercial outcomes argue that, in broad terms, they do so in the following manner. Where the supplier is dominant, it is said that it will take a majority of the surplus value as producer surplus. An example of this might be the relationships between Microsoft® (in its pomp) and its industrial customers. Where the buying organisation is dominant, by contrast, it is said that it will take a majority of the surplus value as consumer surplus. Here, an example could be the big retail supermarkets in their relationships with most food growers. It is said that this will also be the outcome in situations of independence, as there are many buyers and many sellers in such situations. Examples would be markets for stationery, furniture and other low-value organisational purchases. Finally, where there is interdependence, the surplus value is said to be shared. Such scenarios are often seen in the aerospace sector, where there are consolidated markets at many stages of the supply chain. Similar outcomes, in terms of the sharing of surplus value, are said to occur in collaborative relationships that increase the surplus value in the relationship, except that in situations of independence, collaboration will often not be attractive to either party (Cox et al, 2000).

As buyer–supplier power will often affect commercial outcomes, the impact of the concept on procurement practice will be revisited later in the chapter. However, it is important to state at this stage that there is no natural law that says that buyer–supplier power relations *must* affect commercial outcomes in the manner described above – parties to buyer–supplier interactions have agency, after all. It is perfectly possible for parties on the buy-and-sell side to set aside ephemeral or even enduring power advantages, either out of moral conviction or for more calculative reasons, and focus in a different way on serving end-customer or, in this context, patient needs. Indeed, although it goes in some respects beyond the remit of the chapter, there is arguably a strong case for this in areas of highly complex clinical care.

The UK government has over the past 20 years invoked neoclassical (or mainstream) economics in support of its policies. However, there is much to be said for the argument that neoclassical economics are too limited to be used effectively to analyse options for health and social care policy (Lunt et al, 1996; Rice, 1997). As Forder et al (2005, p 98) comment, 'Markets appear to perform well when there is potential for high competition, investments do not tie providers to specific purchasers, complexity and uncertainty are relatively low and/or few scale economies apply. But these are not, arguably, characteristics of health care.' Indeed, nor are they of social care. Accordingly, it has been argued that other schools of thought within economics are better equipped to cope with the complexities of health and social care, in particular transaction cost economics (TCE) (Williamson, 1985).

TCE is based on the aforementioned concept of 'opportunism', but can also be used to make a general point about buyer–supplier power relations. TCE argues that where transactions involve the two parties making considerable transaction-specific investments (for example in equipment, skills or buildings), any competitive tension that the buying organisation was able to bring to bear during the pre-contract negotiations will disappear once the contract begins. This is because the transaction-specific investments cause a 'fundamental transformation', whereby one or both parties find exit from the relationship expensive and time-consuming (Williamson, 1985; see also Chapter Eight, this volume). This is said to have the potential to cause contractual difficulties, especially where uncertainty has led to contractual incompleteness. Uncertainty and contractual incompleteness occur in many large government procurements, for example in the defence sector for weapons systems and in the case of major information technology projects. In such procurements, contracts are often for many years, involve partially developed technologies and concern public sector requirements that change radically and unpredictably over the course of a lengthy contract period. In such circumstances, it is beyond the capabilities of managers, however knowledgeable and experienced, to create a complete contract. This means post-contractual negotiation over changes, which can often be challenging.

Responses suggested by TCE to such a situation, assuming it is not feasible or desirable to reduce the transaction-specific investments, include the integration of the buyer and supplier (in situations where there are no offsetting economies of scale to be obtained from market relations) and the creation of an alliance (in situations where there are still some offsetting scale economies to be gained from keeping the transaction in the marketplace). In the case of an alliance, the buyer and supplier are advised to commit themselves, through the making of joint investments or the posting of 'hostages' (financial bonds or liability arrangements), to a long-term relationship whereby decisions are taken jointly by two mutually dependent organisations (Williamson, 1985). They are then advised to ignore any temporary power advantages that might accrue to them during the contract period and focus on protecting the integrity of the relationship in which they have invested heavily.

These responses of TCE to complexity, uncertainty and transaction-specific investments run, to some degree, contrary to the ideology underpinning UK government health and social care policy for most of the past 20 years. However, while internal integration also has its downsides (as we have already seen), while the threat of opportunism must always be borne in mind (alliances, for example, can become one-sided) and while alliance partners must be selected carefully (see later in the chapter), one of these two responses of TCE may well be the most economically advantageous option in some of the most complex areas of health and social care provision and, in the case of alliances, is, ironically, what private sector organisations are increasingly doing in a whole range of business sectors (Webb and Hughes, 2009). Indeed, the concept of 'integrated care' would appear to be sympathetic to this argument (Ham et al, 2003), although some have argued further that the positive experience in the United States (US) in this respect is not directly replicable in the UK (Lewis and Dixon, 2005).

Managerial responses

Having considered two key behavioural questions related to supplier selection and management, it is now necessary to consider what they mean for procurement practice. In this subsection, therefore, we take the behavioural principles discussed and, with the assistance of examples from the UK health and social care sectors, show how they might affect procurement practice.

Market search and supplier selection

In its assessment of NHS commissioning, Ernst & Young (2009) identified market search, analysis and management as an area of weakness. This view was echoed by Brereton and Vasoodaven (2010, p 29), who commented 'PCTs often lack the ability or resources to purchase effectively and bring about intended benefits for the health system.' Other reports, such as that of Gershon (2004), have contended that these weaknesses extend all across the UK public sector. In this subsection, in response to the criticisms, we look at two issues related to this stage of the procurement process that are critical to achieving best VFM.

While research has demonstrated the advantages of trust (Chiles and McMakin, 1996), few argue that buyers should trust suppliers immediately or unconditionally. Therefore, particularly when procuring certain goods or services for the first time or when dealing with certain suppliers for the first time (but arguably beyond that), buyers are advised to act with caution and accept that they could face either opportunism or the exploitation of power. During the stages in the process concerning search and selection, two hazards in particular require attention. The first is adverse selection (Akerlof, 1970). This is defined as the act of a buyer purchasing a good or service from a supplier at a particular price on the basis that it contains a particular level of quality, when in actual fact (and known to the supplier) it contains (or the intention is for it to contain) a lower level of quality. The result is that the supplier earns an information rent (or abnormal profit) from the deception.

Adverse selection is possible and common in both business and consumer markets, and is a huge issue in relation to health insurance, because, while it is relatively easy in the case of some goods and services to assess the quality of a supplier's offering prior to purchase, in others it is more of a challenge. Indeed, marketers divide goods and services into three 'information categories': search, experience and credence goods (and services) (Mitra et al, 1999). Search goods are those whose quality can be assessed prior to purchase and are usually basic commodity items such as clothing or simple components. Experience goods, including tangible services such as cleaning, have to be consumed before an assessment can be made on quality. Credence goods, meanwhile, which very much include medical procedures, as well as other services such as management consultancy, are those that can be hard for a buyer to assess either pre or post consumption. Adverse selection is a risk in the latter two categories – assuming that the supplier is prepared to act opportunistically.

Given that many public services fall into the experience, and even credence, categories, it is not surprising that opportunism has been mentioned as a potential hazard within health and social care commissioning. Forder et al (2005, p 91) comment 'The quality of health care, particularly in terms of outcomes, is difficult to measure and therefore to write into contracts; purchasers may simply not know [ex ante] whether the services provided are of good quality.' Therefore, where opportunism on the part of suppliers is considered to be a distinct possibility, the search and selection stages of the procurement process for public services will often need to include mechanisms for dealing with adverse selection.

The literature suggests a number of such mechanisms (Milgrom and Roberts, 1992). First, it is suggested that buying organisations consider a remuneration schedule that is based on performance. Second, it suggests warranties, trial periods and short contract periods. Third, it suggests using the threat of contingent renewal – that is, the practice of suggesting to suppliers the possibility of future business, but only if initial goods or performance are acceptable. Fourth, the use of brand reputation is suggested, although there are clear dangers to this. Fifth, it is suggested that buying organisations obtain testimonies from other customers of the supplier. Sixth, in the case of services, it is suggested that buying organisations establish exactly who within the supplier organisation is to provide the service – the problem of the high-quality sales team being replaced during the contract by a lower-quality delivery team is common.

The second issue at the search and selection stage concerns buyer–supplier power. If buyer–supplier power matters to commercial outcomes, and the evidence suggests that buying organisations will often, if not always, be facing suppliers that do indeed intend using power advantages when they have them, then the concept needs to be incorporated into any supplier selection methodology (Cox et al, 2000). This will particularly be in those areas of expenditure where collaborative alliances are sought – certain suppliers will simply not be prepared to forego power advantages and trying to manage alliances with very powerful suppliers that exploit their power can be very difficult, time-consuming and somewhat unrewarding (although sometimes buying organisations are in situations where they have no alternative to trying to make such alliances work) (Ramsay, 1996; Cox, 2005).

A key point here is that even in markets that are quite competitive, it is important to undertake buyer–supplier power analysis. As power is a relative concept, it is likely that even in competitive markets the buying organisation will be in different power positions with different suppliers. This is because, even though all suppliers will face competition in such a market, they will not all equally value the business being offered by the buying organisation. In short, some suppliers will be keener to obtain the buying organisation's business than others (Cox et al, 2000). Indeed, such keen suppliers *may* be a more preferable selection option than other suppliers, even if they are currently less competent in terms of their processes, goods and services. This is because such suppliers may be more amenable to development in directions that are of interest and benefit to the buying organisation and because that development may also allow buyers to fulfil a longer-term objective of developing the supply market concerned.

The fact that buyer–supplier power is a relative concept also re-emphasises the need for effective internal demand management (for example not highly fragmenting demand) and makes it likely that the NHS, as with the rest of the UK public sector, will continue to be interested in the potential of collaborative procurement initiatives (Moffatt, 2010). The grouping together of the demand of a number of public sector bodies, for example groups of PCTs or health and social care joint commissioners, is not a panacea, risks remoteness on the part of commissioners (Smith et al, 2004; House of Commons Health Committee, 2005) and can be difficult to organise, but can in some circumstances increase the utility of the purchase in the eyes of suppliers and deliver results. It certainly seems something worth considering in terms of the commissioning of acute care, given the dominant market position of many acute hospitals.

Suffice to say, adding the concept of 'power' to supplier selection methodologies, admittedly not straightforward (although not impossible) in public procurement because of the EU procurement rules, reveals the selection decision as a trade-off between the ability of a supplier to deliver best VFM and their inclination to do so.

Negotiating with providers

The perspective that buyers have on the behavioural inclinations of suppliers should also colour approaches to negotiation. Ideally (although not, perhaps, in the case of low-value, one-off purchases), buyers should seek to promote 'mutual gains', both in the pre-contractual negotiations and in negotiations during the contractual period (Kinnaird and Movius, 2008). To this end, many frameworks have been developed that encourage buyer and supplier organisations to understand the interests of each party, mutually exploit areas of common interest and creatively find solutions to those areas where there are conflicts of interest (Fisher et al, 1991; Kinnaird and Movius, 2008).

However, where opportunism is feared, such an approach will need to be pursued with caution. A number of hazards present themselves when dealing with potentially opportunistic negotiation counterparts. The first hazard is strategic misrepresentation, or 'bluffing', about positions (Milgrom and Roberts, 1992). During the procurement process the surplus value is divided between the two parties. It has been established that economics defines surplus value as the gap between the buying organisation's utility and the supplier's costs of production. What mainstream economics further assumes, however, is that during negotiations both parties are aware of those two points. This is not, of course, by any means always the case and both parties will often go to great lengths to 'bluff' about such matters, not least as the initial 'anchoring' of the negotiation can have a lasting effect on the outcome.

This strategic misrepresentation might be part of a broader attempt by a negotiation counterpart to employ 'conditioning', that is, the practice of shaping the expectations and perceptions of the other party. Such broader conditioning on the part of a supplier could relate to the general economic or business sector climate, the attractiveness and magnitude of other business options, the relative importance of the buying organisation's business and the discretion that the counterpart has been given by their superiors. Conditioning may also be employed in combination with well-versed non-verbal communication. Sales people are taught both how to present themselves and how to recognise the movements and gestures of their counterparts. The use of the hands and facial gestures are said to be particularly revealing (Collett, 2003).

The possibility of bluffing, conditioning and non-verbal tactics requires buying organisations to carefully select staff members for critical negotiations, ensure that those staff members receive extensive training and, crucially, provide them with the necessary time to both properly prepare and bargain. Many reports into public procurement over the years have commented on the problem of public sector bodies being 'outwitted' by their negotiation counterparts, something that has frequently led to poor VFM outcomes (PAC, 2007; NAO, 2009). Accordingly, cutbacks in this area will often represent a false economy.

A further common problem faced by buying organisations, particularly when they are negotiating complex, long-term contracts with opportunistic suppliers, is pre-contractual drift – that is, the practice of the supplier agreeing to certain concessions during the competitive process, but then seeking to re-open negotiations regarding such concessions when it has been elevated to the position of preferred bidder (Lonsdale and Watson, 2007). Buying organisations are particularly vulnerable to the problem of drift when the preferred bidder selection is made when contractual arrangements are still some way from being finalised. This is because the more time that elapses after the selection of the preferred bidder, the less likely it is that the buying organisation will want to go back and re-open the competition. This will particularly be the case when that organisation is facing a tight deadline, which is often the case in the health and social care sectors. Managers need to consider, therefore, the optimum time of preferred bidder selection and also resist time pressure from the wider organisation.

Therefore, judgement is required in order to assess the balance that should be taken in negotiations between collaborative problem solving and more cautious and defensive actions. Of course, before any of this, the buying team needs to make sure that it arrives at the negotiation with the necessary clinical and commercial information and this, as we have seen, is something that is widely reported to be missing in many public service commercial encounters (House of Commons Health Committee, 2010).

Contractual protection

One of the purposes, of course, of buyer–supplier negotiations is the development of some form of contractual arrangement. As with other stages of the procurement process, the actions of the buying organisation here need to be in line with expectations of supplier behaviour. Where suppliers are trusted to operate in a manner that will promote mutual gains, then contractual incompleteness and dependence will not be seen as a cause for concern. Economists have variously called such a relaxed approach 'general clause' or 'relational' contracting (Macneil, 1978; Williamson, 1985) and have pointed to the lower transaction costs and greater flexibility that accompanies such an approach (Chiles and McMakin, 1996).

However, where opportunism is feared, it is argued that buying organisations should use pre-contract negotiations to craft greater contractual protection, even at the cost of some of the benefits of a more relaxed approach. First, buying organisations are advised, where possible, to specify clearly, accurately and comprehensively, having come to the negotiating table well informed. Second, buying organisations are advised to create a series of contractual incentives. Incentives are said to be required in order to discourage moral hazard. Moral hazard arises when the actions of one party (in the current context, the service provider) are hidden and the incentives in the relationship are misaligned, that is, one party stands to gain from not acting in the interests of the other party, albeit in a manner that does not break the letter of the contract (Milgrom and Roberts, 1992). Whether moral hazard is a feasible option for a supplier depends on the level of supplier discretion that characterises either production or service delivery. Where supplier moral hazard is feasible, buying organisations are advised to realign the incentives by, for example, linking payments to service levels and delivery milestones, establishing penalties and creating gain-share arrangements. They are also advised to back up such measures with a system of monitoring and to use the tactic of contingent renewal.

Numerous examples of moral hazard within the commissioning arena can be provided. The ending of block contracts for acute care was, of course, in part, intended to address perceived moral hazard. It was, and is, hoped that Payment by Results will eradicate the complacency apparently encouraged by block contracts. The practice of 'up-coding', that is, unjustifiably recording the most expensive diagnosis under the Payment by Results tariff system (Mannion and Street, 2009), is a further example of moral hazard (see Box 4.3); as is provider-induced demand, another problem thought to have been an unintended consequence of Payment by Results. Brereton and Vasoodaven (2010, p 9) explain this latter example: '[Acute hospitals] being paid per case through Payment by Results produces adverse incentives for hospitals to increase activity beyond affordable levels and possibly induce demand inappropriately'.

Box 4.3: Case example: 'up-coding' as an example of potential moral hazard

While providers deny practicing 'up-coding', the logic of it under Payment by Results is clear, particularly if providers are facing financial pressures. The King's Fund comments in relation to heart attack treatment:

> [H]ospitals can start to cheat on coding. For instance, the NHS tariff pays two prices for different kinds of heart attack treatment: £1775 for treatment of patients without medical complications and £3676 for those with complications. The risk is that hospitals will falsify the code (or worse still give unnecessary treatment) in order to make more money.

Source: King's Fund (2005, p 3)

Indeed, great care needs to be taken over the setting of incentives, because of this problem of unintended consequences. Mannion and Davies (2008, p 307) comment 'If the reward is small the effect may be negligible. Conversely, large incentives may lead to major, potentially unpredictable, changes. As rewards rise, so do the risks of adverse consequences. Responses may also be influenced by whether the performance payments are a potential gain or a potential loss.' An example of the concerns expressed about incentive schemes is provided by Commissioning for Quality and Innovation (CQUIN), the NHS financial incentive related to quality outcomes. There is a fear it may destabilise providers, increase tension between commissioners and providers, while at the same time not being particularly effective in improving quality. Maynard and Bloor (2010, p 298) comment 'Experience from the US suggests that a balance needs to be struck between the motivational effects of potential penalties and the possible costs of destabilising organisations. In addition, if penalties are a real possibility and are on occasion levied, their motivational effects are likely to be short-lived.'

Third, and particularly in the case of complex and large-scale purchases or projects containing significant transaction-specific investments, buying organisations are advised to consider using the contract to create 'contractual balance' or interdependence, as part of a broader attempt to create an alliance. The idea behind this is that, as discussed earlier in the chapter, it will provide the motivation for mutual cooperation, problem solving and innovation. One way of achieving this interdependence is said to be through joint investment. For example, if there are transaction-specific investments that need to be made in the relationship, it is suggested that efforts are made so that both parties incur part of such investment. If this happens, then it is said that both parties will have an incentive to refrain from opportunistic actions as both will have an interest in protecting the transaction-specific investments they have made (Williamson, 1985). Where that is not possible, and it is inevitable that the transaction-specific investments will cause one party to be dependent, it is suggested that one party posts 'hostages' (in the aforementioned form of financial bonds or liability arrangements) in order to contrive balance (Williamson, 1985). This type of contractual protection has worked well elsewhere in the UK public sector (NAO, 2003) and might be suitable for the aforementioned integrated health and social care delivery initiatives.

Contract management

Contract management, broadly speaking, consists of monitoring, measurement and supplier relationship management (SRM). Once again, the view taken about likely supplier behaviour, as well as the size and/or importance of the expenditure, will affect the balance between them. When opportunism is feared, the focus will be on monitoring and performance measurement, to either guard against the aforementioned moral hazard or simply to ensure basic contractual fulfilment. As indicated earlier in the chapter, any performance system needs to be carefully designed. Performance indicators, whether they are compiled by the buyer or supplier, need to possess credibility (Mannion and Goddard, 2001) and performance regimes need to take account of the potential for unintended and dysfunctional consequences (Mannion and Davies, 2008). Where suppliers are believed to be of more trustworthy intent, either through a bold initial assessment or following a period of confidence-building interaction, buying organisations can more extensively link performance measurement to performance improvement (Hughes, 2005). The mechanism here is SRM, a blanket term used to cover a whole range of activities that buying organisations can undertake, particularly within an alliance, in order to increase the surplus value in a relationship.

This range of activities, aimed at enhancing goods and services or reducing cost, can be placed within a number of categories. These are:

- product and process information exchange;
- operational linkages (for example 'just-in-time' systems and vendor-managed inventory arrangements);
- cooperative norms (for example dispute resolution channels or trust-enhancing events);
- transaction-specific investments (Cannon and Perreault, 1999).

SRM is presented as a necessary development as it is argued that the gains from sourcing more effectively, for example through the adoption of category management and the additional competitive leverage that often results from its adoption, will quite quickly deliver diminishing returns, as supplier margins can only be reduced so far. SRM is presented as a way of the procurement process continuing to deliver improved VFM, and in ways that are of greater long-term value to the organisation than simple cost savings.

The gains of SRM have to be earned, however, through organisational commitment and discipline. One of the reasons why many SRM programmes fail is that insufficient resources are committed to their implementation. For example, SRM tasks are often given to managers with an already full workload, causing such tasks to be neglected. Another cause of failure is that even where a full-time supplier relationship manager is appointed, that person is undermined by other managers and internal stakeholders bombarding the supplier with contradictory messages, priorities and demands (Webb and Hughes, 2009). There are echoes of this in the recent House of Commons Health Committee (2010) report into healthcare commissioning, which identified a poor level of provider relationship management and a failure to engage in constructive performance dialogue in order to promote ongoing quality improvements.

Of course, when we are discussing SRM (perhaps as part of an attempt to create a close alliance with a supplier), we are again, to some extent, contradicting the message of the UK market reforms that encourage the creation of competitive tension. Not that SRM should be mistaken for a soft option. What SRM does reject, however, is the idea that competition tension is necessary at all times for performance improvement and may be appropriate to a number of health and social care purchasing circumstances.

Case study in internal and external management

Therefore, there is a whole range of internal and external supply market issues that commissioners need to address if they are to achieve best VFM. Commissioners must also recognise the connection between internal and external supply market actions. In order to illustrate and draw together much of the discussion in this chapter on these matters, a case is provided from another part of the UK public sector. It concerns National Savings and Investments (NS&I) and the outsourcing of its business operations to a private sector supplier (see Box 4.4). The case shows how seriously NS&I took its internal preparations and management (including that of managing political expectations) and shows how this made it easier for the organisation to deal effectively with the supply market. As can be seen, the opportunity created was not squandered. No procurement exercise is perfect and this is no exception. However, it does provide a good example of an organisation heeding the messages of the economics presented in this chapter.

Box 4.4: Case example: NS&I

In 1997, NS&I, a financial institution operating out of the UK public sector, outsourced its business operations. This included all operational tasks and processes, except the design and marketing of its financial products. NS&I wanted to keep such tasks in-house as they are necessary for the public sector to control the policy direction of the organisation.

In addition to this in-sourcing decision, NS&I made three other key internal decisions. First, it carefully created a team with broad expertise and experience, mindful of the many occasions in which the public sector had been remiss in preparation for and 'outwitted' in negotiations. The team included operational, commercial and senior managers from NS&I and external consultants from HM Treasury and private sector organisations. Second, considerable time and care was taken to ensure that the proposal to be taken into the marketplace both satisfied internal stakeholders and represented a credible commercial and technical proposition for providers. Third, time was taken over the negotiations, with political pressure for a rapid settlement resisted.

Having prepared the ground internally, NS&I then sent out its call for proposals. This prompted nearly 100 responses, of which four were shortlisted. These bidders developed their proposals, with EDS and Siemens Business Services (SBS) winning through to the last round. At this point, NS&I decided to extend the competition between EDS and SBS until it had negotiated a draft contract with both parties. This was to avoid the problem of pre-contractual drift. Eventually, a decision was made to award the contract to SBS.

The following contractual arrangement was agreed with SBS:

- SBS was to be responsible for all operational tasks required to deliver NS&I savings products.
- SBS agreed to reduce its operational costs year on year during the contract.
- The management of new NS&I products was to be opened up to competition if SBS's performance was deemed unacceptable by NS&I.
- SBS was obliged to help with any transition to another supplier.
- A formal change process was agreed to deal with the inevitable uncertainty surrounding the contract.
- NS&I was to share in SBS profits, where deemed excessive.
- SBS was solely responsible under the contract for operational errors.
- A wide-ranging set of key performance indicators was agreed.
- A monitoring system was agreed.

Underpinning all of this was a further agreement that SBS's parent company would guarantee its obligations under the contract. Its liability, triggered not least if SBS walked away from the contract, was set at £250 million. This had the effect of balancing the relationship and making the other contractual arrangements enforceable. After all, NS&I was making itself totally dependent on SBS and, while it retained the right to switch suppliers, such a switch would be a last resort, given the time and money it would cost NS&I. Without the liability provision, SBS might have been tempted to exploit the dependency during the course of the contract, especially if it is was not achieving its hoped-for returns.

In 2003, the National Audit Office reported that both operationally and commercially the contract had been successful in its first five years.

Source: Adapted from NAO (2003)

Conclusion

This chapter has provided an overview of the core principles and practices related to procurement and supply management. It provides a starting point for readers, who are encouraged to use the list of references to immerse themselves further in what is a fascinating, divided and diverse theoretical literature. What the chapter has also provided is evidence that this theoretical literature is of relevance to the UK health and social care system. While many features of the UK health and social care system are unique (indeed, some are very unique), there are also many other features, such as internal politics, tight markets, dominant providers and supplier opportunism, that can be seen anywhere in either the public or the private sector. The literature can be used to analyse such problems and suggest responses.

To this end, there have been a number of key messages in the chapter. The first is that successful procurement processes start inside the buying organisation. Effective internal demand management is critical to the overall effectiveness of any procurement exercise, although not always easily secured. The second is that it is necessary to consider the nature of the behavioural environment, internally and externally, before deciding on practical ways forward. Managers must consider the political sensitivity of any procurement exercise and also consider the likely behaviour of the suppliers it will come into contact with – otherwise, they may receive some unwelcome surprises.

The third message, partly as a result of the second, is that managers involved in procurement need to adopt a contingency approach – that is, match their actions to the specific nature of the purchase in question. For example, on some occasions, arm's-length, adversarial contracting will be appropriate. On others, more engaged approaches with suppliers will be preferable. On others still, 'in-sourcing', or vertical integration, will be the best option. The right choice will depend on a number of factors, including the size of the purchase, its importance, uncertainty, current performance levels, power relations and expected supplier behaviour. Managers should approach a purchase without prejudice and calculate the best way forward. Of course, whether in the UK health and social care market, managers will always be allowed to do this, is another matter.

Further reading

- Further discussion of the ideas presented in this chapter can be found in Cox, A., Lonsdale, C., Sanderson, J., Watson, G. and Ireland, P. (2003) *Supply chain management: a guide to best practice*, London: Financial Times and Prentice Hall.
- For a more general text on procurement and supply management, readers may wish to access Cousins, P., Lamming, R., Lawson, B. and Squire, B. (2007) *Strategic supply management*, London: Financial Times and Prentice Hall.
- A good journal for managers is *CPO Agenda*, which sits in between trade and academic journals in the area. *Procurement Leaders* is also a useful source.
- Those seeking academic studies on the subject, however, could look at the *Journal of Purchasing and Supply Management, Supply Chain Management: An International Journal* and the *Journal of Public Procurement*.

Useful websites

Organisation	Outline of available resources	Website
Audit Commission	Online reports of past procurement and market management activity in the NHS and UK public sector more generally	www.audit-commission.gov.uk/
Chartered Institute of Purchasing & Supply (CIPS)	Website of the UK professional body that serves procurement professionals in the UK and beyond. Site contains a wide range of 'professional resources', including guidance on practice	www.cips.org/
Department of Health	Official government website providing guidance on NHS policy and practice in relation to procurement	www.dh.gov.uk/
House of Commons Health Committee	Online reports of past procurement and market management activity in the NHS	www.parliament.uk/
National Audit Office	Online reports of past procurement and market management activity in the NHS and UK public sector more generally	www.nao.org.uk/
Spend Matters UK/Europe	Expert 'blog-site', run by a former president of CIPS, that discusses the latest developments in purchasing and market management, especially in the UK public sector	www.spendmatters.co.uk/

Reflective exercises

1. To what extent do you believe that your organisation matches the description given of a 'political organisation'? To what extent does this affect commissioning? How might your organisation use the idea of organisations being 'political' to solve internal problems that affect commissioning outcomes?

2. To what extent do you believe that you encounter 'opportunistic' provider behaviour? What specific types of 'opportunism' are most common? What mechanisms does your organisation use to deal with them? How do you believe that 'opportunistic' provider behaviour can best be addressed?

3. Do you believe that purchaser–provider power relations matter to commissioning outcomes? Where your organisation is suffering from adverse power relations with providers, how easy do you believe it is to rebalance those relations? How can you rebalance those relations?

4. What are the advantages and disadvantages of the purchaser–provider split? What alternatives are there to the split and how might they work?

References

Akerlof, G. (1970) 'The market for "lemons": quality uncertainty and the market mechanism', *The Quarterly Journal of Economics*, vol 83, no 4, pp 488-500.

Bartlett, W. and Le Grand, J. (1993) 'The theory of quasi-markets', in J. Le Grand and W. Bartlett (eds) *Quasi-markets and social policy*, Basingstoke: Macmillan, pp 13-34.

Brereton, L. and Vasoodaven, V. (2010) *The impact of the NHS market: an overview of the literature*, London: Civitas.

Burnes, B. and Pope, R. (2007) 'Negative behaviours in the workplace: a study of two primary care trusts in the NHS', *International Journal of Public Sector Management*, vol 20, no 4, pp 285-303.

Cannon, J. and Perreault, W. (1999) 'Buyer–seller relationships in business markets', *Journal of Marketing Research*, vol 36, no 4, pp 439-60.

Chiles, T. and McMakin, J. (1996) 'Integrating variable risk preferences, trust, and transaction cost economics', *Academy of Management Review*, vol 21, no 1, pp 73-99.

Collett, P. (2003) *The book of tells*, London: Bantam.

Cox, A. (2005) 'The problem with win-win', *CPO Agenda*, autumn, available online via www.cpoagenda.org

Cox, A., Sanderson, J. and Watson, G. (2000) *Power regimes*, Boston, MA: Earlsgate Press.

Cross, M. (2010) 'Commissioning a bridge for GP's information gap', *Smarthealthcare.com*, 18 August, www.smarthealthcare.com

DCLG (Department for Communities and Local Government) (2008) *The national procurement strategy for local government: final report*, London: DCLG.

DH (Department of Health) (2007) *World class commissioning: vision*, London: DH.

DH (2010) *Equity and excellence: liberating the NHS*, London: TSO.

Ellinor, R. (2007) 'Engaging change', *Supply Management*, 19 July, www.supplymanagement.com

Emerson, R. (1962) 'Power-dependence relations', *American Sociological Review*, vol 27, no 1, pp 31-41.

Ernst & Young (2009) *Understanding health care markets: a PCT guide to market analysis and market management*, London: Ernst & Young.

Fisher, R., Ury, W. and Patton, B. (1991) *Getting to yes*, London: Random House.

Forder, J., Robinson, R. and Hardy, B. (2005) 'Theoretical perspectives on purchasing', in J. Figueras, R. Robinson and E. Jakubowski (eds) *Purchasing to improve health systems performance*, Buckingham: Open University Press, pp 83-101.

Freidson, E. (1986) *Professional powers: a study of the institutionalization of formal knowledge*, Chicago, IL : University of Chicago Press.

French, J. and Raven, B. (1959) 'Bases of social power', in D. Cartwright (ed) *Studies in social power*, Ann Arbor, MI: University of Michigan Press, pp 150-67.

Gershon, P. (2004) *Releasing resources to the front line: independent review of public sector efficiency*, London: HM Treasury.

Gilbert, H. (2007) 'Gun control', *Supply Management*, 15 March, www.supplymanagement.com

Ham, C., York, N., Sutch, S. and Shaw, R. (2003) 'Hospital bed utilisation in the NHS, Kaiser Permanente, and the US Medicare programme: analysis of routine data', *British Medical Journal*, vol 327, pp 1257-60.

Hawkins, D. (2010) 'A question of trust', *Supply Management*, www.supplymanagement.com

Hay, C. (2007) *Why we hate politics*, Cambridge: Polity Press.

Hickson, D., Hinings, C., Lee, C., Schneck, R. and Pennings, J. (1971) 'A strategic contingencies theory of intraorganizational power', *Administrative Science Quarterly*, vol 16, no 2, pp 216-29.

House of Commons Health Committee (2005) *Changes to primary care trusts*, London: TSO.

House of Commons Health Committee (2010) *Commissioning*, London: TSO.

Hughes, J. (2005) 'Supplier metrics that matter', *CPO Agenda*, autumn, pp 19-23.

Hughes, J., Ralf, M. and Michels, B. (1998) *Transform your supply chain*, London: International Thompson Business Press.

King's Fund (2005) *Payment by results*, London: King's Fund.

Kinnaird, T. and Movius, H. (2008) 'Avoiding the three deadly sins', *CPO Agenda*, autumn, www.cpoagenda.org

Lewis, R. and Dixon, J. (2005) *The future of primary care: meeting the challenges of the new NHS market*, London: King's Fund.

Lonsdale, C. and Watson, G. (2005) 'The internal client relationship, demand management and value for money: a conceptual model', *Journal of Purchasing and Supply Management*, vol 11, no 5, pp 159-72.

Lonsdale, C. and Watson, G. (2007) 'Managing contracts under the Private Finance Initiative', *Policy & Politics*, vol 35, no 4, pp 683-700.

Lukes, S. (1974) *Power: a radical view*, New York, NY: Free Press.

Lunt, N., Mannion, R. and Smith, P. (1996) 'Economic discourse and the market: the case of community care', *Public Administration*, vol 74, no 3, pp 369-91.

Macneil, I. (1978) 'Contracts: adjustment of long-term economic relations under classical, neoclassical and relational contract law', *Northwestern University Law Review*, vol 72, no 6, pp 854-905.

Mannion, R. and Davies, H. (2008) 'Payment for performance in health care', *British Medical Journal*, vol 336, pp 306-8.

Mannion, R. and Goddard, M. (2001) 'Impact of published clinical outcomes data: case study in NHS hospital trusts', *British Medical Journal*, vol 323, pp 260-3.

Mannion, R. and Street, A. (2009) 'Managing activity and expenditure in the new NHS', *Public Money & Management*, vol 29, no 1, pp 27-34.

Mannion, R., Davies, H. and Marshall, M. (2005) *Cultures for performance in health care*, Maidenhead: Open University Press.

March, J. (1994) *A primer on decision making*, New York, NY: Free Press.

Mayer, R., Davis, J. and Schoorman, F. (1995) 'An integrative model of organizational trust', *Academy of Management Review*, vol 20, no 3, pp 709-34.

Maynard, A. and Bloor, K. (2010) 'Will financial incentives and penalties improve hospital care?', *British Medical Journal*, vol 340, pp 297-8.

Milgrom, P. and Roberts, J. (1992) *Economics, organization and management*, New York, NY: Prentice Hall.

Mitra, K., Reiss, M. and Capella, L. (1999) 'An examination of perceived risk, information search and behavioural intentions in search, experience and credence services', *The Journal of Services Marketing*, vol 13, no 3, pp 208-28.

Moffatt, S. (2010) 'Uniform approach to police savings', *Supply Management*, 15 April, www.supplymanagement.com

NAO (National Audit Office) (2003) *National Savings and Investments' deal with Siemens Business Services: four years on*, London: NAO.

NAO (2009) *Commercial skills for complex government projects*, London: NAO.

Nooteboom, B. (2002) *Trust*, Cheltenham: Edward Elgar.

PAC (Public Accounts Committee) (2003) *New IT systems for magistrates' courts: the Libra project – examination of witnesses*, London: PAC.

PAC (2007) *Update on PFI debt refinancing and the PFI equity market: press notice*, 15 May, London: PAC.

Pettigrew, A. (1977) 'Strategy formulation as a political process', *International Studies of Management and Organizations*, vol 7, no 2, pp 78-87.

Pfeffer, J. (1981) *Power in organizations*, Marshfield, MA: Pitman.

Ramsay, J. (1996) 'The case against purchasing partnerships', *Journal of Supply Chain Management*, vol 32, no 4, pp 13-19.

Rice, T. (1997) 'Can markets give us the health system we want?', *Journal of Health Politics, Policy and Law*, vol 22, no 2, pp 383-426.

Robinson, P., Faris, C. and Wind, Y. (1967) *Industrial buying behaviour and creative marketing*, Boston, MA: Allyn & Bacon.

Russill, R. (2003) 'The clan strikes back', *Supply Management*, 8 May, pp 24-5.

Simon, H. (1957) *Models of man*, New York, NY: Wiley.

Smith, J., Mays, N., Dixon, J., Goodwin, N., Lewis, R., McClelland, S., McLeod, H. and Wyke, S. (2004) *A review of the effectiveness of primary-care led commissioning and its place in the NHS*, London: The Health Foundation.

Smith, P. (2003) 'Return to centre', *Supply Management*, 10 April 10, pp 20-4.

Smith, P. (2009) 'On your marks', *Supply Management*, 22 October, www.supplymanagement.com

Webb, M. and Hughes, J. (2009) 'Building the case for SRM', *CPO Agenda*, autumn, pp 46-50.

Williamson, O. (1985) *The economic institutions of capitalism*, New York, NY: Free Press.

Williamson, O. (1996) *Mechanisms of governance*, Oxford: Oxford University Press.

FIVE

Decommissioning services

Ray Puffitt and Lesley Prince

Summary

This chapter explores:
- the importance and traditional neglect of decommissioning;
- possible matrix-based approaches;
- a key framework that health and social care commissioners can use in practice;
- worked examples of the framework in action.

Following the dislocation experienced by the global economy, its impact on the United Kingdom (UK) economy and the consequent financial constraints on public spending, it is likely that many more public services will be decommissioned over the next few years than has been the case in the past. Indeed, decommissioning may well become a central feature of the working life of all public service commissioning and procurement staff. Yet, the decision to decommission a service is always fraught with uncertainty and difficulty, especially when powerful forces support the status quo. In the context of local government, these powerful forces include, inter alia, the elected members who over time may have invested considerable thought, commitment and resources into a particular service, whether provided in-house or procured from the market, and about which they are in consequence somewhat protective.

The decision to decommission a service might well be seen by the workforce, whether highly skilled or not, as a direct devaluing of their contribution to the organisation, perhaps generating resentment as well as anger and anxiety. In other circumstances it might be the service users themselves or other key stakeholders such as external providers, carers, parents, patients, family or neighbours who are fearful that the effects of the decision to decommission will have a detrimental impact on their well-being. Inevitably, this places a considerable burden of practical, moral and above all political responsibility on those managers whose job it is to decide on decommissioning any existing service. In practical terms they will initially need to assess the likely levels and nature of any difficulties that may be generated by the decision to decommission. This will have a direct influence on the rigour with which the recommendation to decommission is put forward, and therefore on the ability to meet any political or legal challenges subsequent to the decision itself, or indeed whether the decision is finally implemented at all. Accordingly, an overall assessment of the context in which the decision to decommission is to be made is essential, and this requires a careful, rigorous and valid consideration of *all* the relevant factors properly weighted. This, of course, is only the beginning of the process, and although rudimentary in these initial stages it will provide not only a clarification of relevant issues, but also an essential audit trail for the final decision itself.

Against this background, this chapter considers an analytical tool capable of being used for such an analysis in both the initial and the subsequent stages of the decision-making process: the Maslin Multi-Dimensional Matrix (MMDM) (Prince and Puffitt, 2001). Decommissioning is such a complex and often neglected task that the focus of the chapter is very much on the practical tools and techniques that commissioners can use when faced with a potentially difficult decommissioning decision. In particular, the chapter offers a detailed worked example of the MMDM in practice, building on this analysis in the subsequent chapter on commissioning for service resilience.

Matrices in decision making

Public servants are familiar with using two-dimensional matrices for structuring and clarifying their thinking and analysis. In recent years, the so-called Value for Money matrix has been used extensively. In principle (although not always in practice) this method is straightforward and relatively easy to use. In a conventional 2 × 2 matrix, cost is plotted against quality and the intersection marked by an X. If the plot falls on a 45° line drawn from the origin, this is said to represent value for money (see Figure 5.1).

In the example given in Figure 5.1, XB represents a high-quality but high-cost service whereas XA represents a low-quality but also low-cost service. Both these services exhibit value for money because in this simple two-dimensional test of cost against quality they both appear on the 45° line. Anything off the line can be interpreted as either exceptional value for money (high quality; low cost) or very poor value for money (high cost; low quality).

Similarly, the Best Value matrix is also a two-dimensional matrix but this time the test is comparative cost versus comparative quality. That is to say, it compares the cost and quality of the service being evaluated against other providers of the

Figure 5.1: The Value for Money matrix

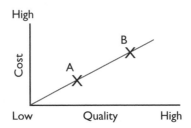

same service. Unlike the Value for Money matrix, however, this matrix is scaled by percentiles (in practice a five-point scale based on quartiles), as shown in Figure 5.2.

Figure 5.2: Best Value matrix

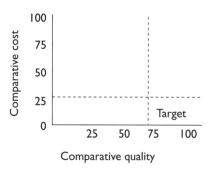

The target is to reach the upper quartile for quality (75th percentile or better) and having identified the upper quartile providers, which quarter of them have the lowest costs. This concept is enshrined in DETR Circular 10/99 (Department of the Environment, Transport and the Regions, 1999), which admittedly only applies statutorily to English local authorities but nevertheless as a concept the term 'Best Value' is common in nearly all UK government official literatures.

The Boston Matrix is another two-dimensional matrix developed by the Boston Consulting Group specifically for marketing purposes, principally within the private sector, and which is exceptionally well known to public servants. However, it suffers from the weaknesses of all two-dimensional matrices when applied to public service commissioning activities as it does not capture the complexity of public services with their multiple competing objectives, concerns and stakeholder groups. Furthermore, the important dimensions of the relationship between a public service and its service users are not usually the two prescribed dimensions of the Boston Matrix, which are 'market share' and 'market growth'. For a detailed, academic critique of the Boston Matrix, the related Montanari Matrix and a theoretical articulation of the MMDM, see Prince and Puffitt (2001).

Accordingly, what is required for rigorous analysis in public services is a multi-dimensional matrix that captures the principal dimensions that mediate the relationship of the service with the political, cultural and social environment in which it is provided.

The MMDM

The fundamental principle behind the MMDM (see Figure 5.3) is what may be called 'creative clarification'; a process of approaching the difficult problem of decommissioning a service (and in the following chapter 'commissioning for service resilience') systematically, but without expelling the creativity essential to sound decision making. It was initially developed by academics at the University of Birmingham's Institute of Local Government Studies seeking to produce a

Figure 5.3: The MMDM

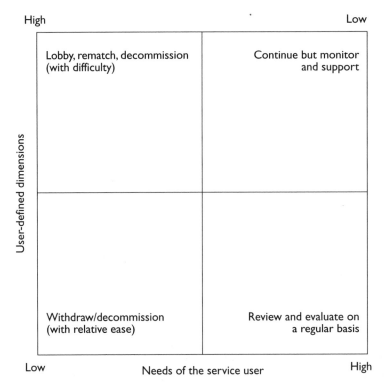

High   Low

Lobby, rematch, decommission (with difficulty)   Continue but monitor and support

User-defined dimensions

Withdraw/decommission (with relative ease)   Review and evaluate on a regular basis

Low   Needs of the service user   High

practical and accessible tool that was theoretically robust – but which could be easily applied in the real world of public service commissioning by busy managers and practitioners.

In public services, quality is assessed, in general terms, by how well a service is matched with the needs of the service user or other key stakeholders so that the primary objectives or outcomes of the service are achieved. Therefore, the central purpose of the MMDM is to identify and clarify the *linkages* between the services that the organisation provides or procures and the important dimensions of the service's relationship with its service users or other stakeholders. Its name is derived from this purpose: *ma*tching *s*ervice *lin*kages. Its primary analysis is an exploration of situations in which there is a *poor* match, which one might describe as exhibiting disequilibrium, tension or turbulence in the relationship; and, on the other hand, where there is a *good* match or, in other words, equilibrium, harmony or stability. Where there is a *poor* match, it indicates the need to lobby and rematch the service so that better outcomes are achieved. Where there is a very high degree of 'mismatch' it will also give a fair indication of the level of difficulty likely to be experienced in making service change.

In its basic form, the MMDM looks similar to most other two–dimensional models: it comprises a 2 × 2 matrix of four cells. However, it differs fundamentally in that while the dimension on the x-axis is predefined as 'needs of the service user', the dimensions on the y-axis are not defined and therefore the analyst is in complete control of what dimensions to include and exclude, what to prioritise and, most importantly, the *interpretation* of the results. Its primary orientation is towards *descriptive* analysis and clarification of situations that are likely to have an important bearing on the final decision. In principle, there may be infinitely many dimensions that define the relationship between a public service and the environment in which it operates, although in practice and from experience using the matrix, there will effectively be between 12 and 15 that most adequately define the decision space, depending on the primary issues that must be taken into account, when decommissioning a service.

X axis: 'needs of the service user'

Derivation of the 'needs of the service user' is extremely important and requires careful clarification. In general, however, the 'needs' of a service user of a public service organisation are laid down in some form of rule, eligibility criteria or code of good practice, whereas 'wants' or expressed demands are simply desires (see also Chapter Two, this volume). Wants exist solely in the mind. One wants a car, a house or the latest fashion and the sole and final arbiter as to whether that want can be satisfied is preparedness and ability to pay the market price, or persuading someone else to meet it on one's behalf. Needs, on the other hand, as understood within public services, are derived from 'rules' of some sort: legal, political or sometimes moral. Obviously, these imply particular sets of values and interests as well.

To illustrate this point, consider the following examples. A person may *want* a house, but if that person is unable to pay the market price, by way of either purchase or rent, then they cannot have a house unless they are able to establish their *need* for a house by satisfying the criteria, as laid down by statute or policy, for the award of social housing or housing benefit and therefore fall within the remit of the appropriate public authorities. If they are unable so to do, they would be judged as having a 'low need for the service as currently provided'.

To take another example, imagine a methadone dosing service that is available 365 days a year, open each day for 18 hours with somewhat sloppy administrative procedures and a very poor rate of recovery. Because of the laxity in procedures there is no serious attempt to prevent 'double-scripting', little notice is taken of the users to prevent them from dealing on the premises, and there is little pressure on the clients to ensure that they stay for counselling for their substance use. From the users' point of view, they may well consider that the service is fine, especially because of its accessibility, and will *want* the service to remain as it is. From the point of view of the authorities, however, clearly it presents a series of problems. Those commissioning the service may well conclude that it does not comply with rules regarding eligibility, good practice and clinical governance, nor is it effectively meeting the legitimate needs of the service user group for which it is intended. As a consequence, action will probably have to be taken; it will need to be reconfigured or decommissioned.

Using these two examples to further illustrate the status of the labels high and low on the x-axis, these evaluations in terms of need are usually set out in formal criteria of some kind. The analyst will have made themselves familiar with such criteria and what is considered to be 'good practice' and, coupled with the monitoring and market intelligence they possess, have come to an initial belief that it may be necessary to decommission the service. The dimension, therefore, for the x-axis becomes (*low*) 'need for the service as currently provided'. Consequently, when considering the decision to decommission a service (as opposed to commissioning for service resilience, which will be explored in the following chapter) the analyst is inevitably considering only the left-hand side of the matrix.

Y-axis: user definitions

The y-axis is purely user defined, according to requirements. By user, we mean the person undertaking the analysis and ultimately producing a report. In a detailed analysis, between 10 and 15 dimensions will be defined, which will be restricted only by what is regarded as salient to the analysis, and naturally different parties may disagree on what is or is not salient. Accordingly, it is clearly not possible to provide an exhaustive or definitive list of the kinds of dimensions that may be used; therefore, the following list provides a representative sample of the principal dimensions that users have deployed in the past when using the matrix:

1. level of staff expertise;
2. level of media interest;
3. level of concern by elected members or other influential parties;
4. level of possibility of redundancies;
5. level of current deployment of resources (land, property, equipment, staff and so on);
6. level of congruence with statutory objectives;
7. level of current providers' 'connective' or political influence;
8. level of 'cartelling' by providers;
9. level of finance expended on the current service;
10. level of implications for other agencies;
11. level of concern by service users;
12. level of concern by other key stakeholders (for example, carers, parents, family, community or others);
13. level of existing monopoly;
14. level of accessibility of current service.

Many of these dimensions, it will be noted, are concerned with bodies other than the one making the decision and this again highlights the principle that in the public sector decisions are often made in the light of another group's concerns and priorities. Some of these bodies also represent a 'higher' authority: national government, 'the market', a professional body, a management team, a trade federation and so on. Moreover, in undertaking the analysis the analyst has to be certain that their 'market intelligence' is sound, that they are fully aware of the concerns of others by undertaking extensive consultation with affected parties and not merely treating the analysis as a desktop exercise divorced from an accurate appreciation of the views of those who may be affected by their recommendations.

The tasks to be undertaken

In undertaking the analysis there are three primary tasks. The first and principal one is to plot the service on the left-hand side of the matrix against, at least, the 14 dimensions outlined earlier.

Task 1: Plot the service

Plot the service above the centre-line or below (see Figure 5.4). By way of illustration, take the example of a day care service for older people. The level of staff expertise is likely to be relatively low, hence dimension 1 is plotted below the centre-line in Figure 5.4. The level of media interest is also likely to be relatively low for this particular category of service user, hence dimension 2 is plotted below the line. The level of concern by elected members is also likely to be low, unless it is a facility provided within their ward (see 3 in Figure 5.4).

Figure 5.4: Practical example I

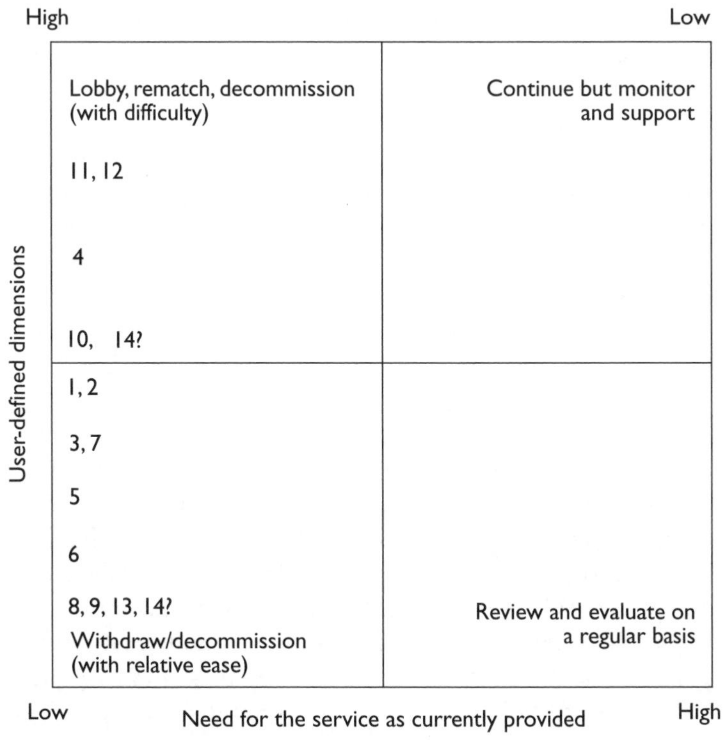

The possibility of redundancies, albeit perhaps that there is only a low number of staff employed, will be high unless they can be redeployed by the provider in some other service or locality (see 4 in Figure 5.4). The current deployment of resources (land, property, equipment and so on) is likely to be relatively insignificant (see 5 in Figure 5.4). The level of congruence with statutory objectives is low as this is a discretionary rather than mandatory service (see 6 in Figure 5.4). The level of the provider's connective or political influence will usually be low unless the service has in the past been championed by a local elected member or other locally prominent person (see 7 in Figure 5.4). It is unlikely that a provider of this type of service would be in a position to 'cartel' the commissioning authority (see 8 in Figure 5.4). With regard to the level of finance expended on the service, the day rate paid will be relatively insignificant and even when multiplied by the number of users will represent only a tiny proportion of the commissioner's budget (see 9 in Figure 5.4). The level of implication for other agencies may, however, be quite significant. For example, general practitioners (GPs) might well experience an increase in referrals to their own services if the day care service is decommissioned (see 10 in Figure 5.4). The level of concern by service users may be very high, especially if no replacement or substitute service is to be provided (see 11 in Figure 5.4). Similarly, the level of concern by other key stakeholders will also be very high as they will lose a facility that provides them with respite (see 12 in Figure 5.4). It is unlikely that the provider will have a high level of monopoly for there may be a multiplicity of other potential providers or substitute ways of meeting the need for social activity and respite (see 13 in Figure 5.4). The level of accessibility of the service will be solely determined by the location of the facility in relation to its principal users – it may be very local, in which case dimension 14 would be plotted high on the matrix, or it may not be, in which case it would be plotted low (see 14 in Figure 5.4).

The implication of this analysis is that with the exception of 4, 10, 11 and 12, it should be fairly easy to withdraw from, that is to say decommission, this particular service. Naturally, in an ideal world the commissioner would attempt to find a way of mitigating the effects on service users, carers, GPs and the staff employed, but the reality may well be that, faced with economic dislocation and financial constraint, other services will be deemed to be of greater priority and therefore the day care service will be decommissioned notwithstanding the difficulties that this may pose.

To take a different example, imagine a voluntary organisation providing residential accommodation for people with severe learning disability where half of the places are commissioned by the local authority and the remaining places are commissioned by other agencies. Some of the members of the management committee of the voluntary organisation are also politically active on the local council, the dedicated GP is chair of the GP commissioning consortium and some of the parents and/or carers are involved with the local media. Furthermore, the voluntary organisation is closely linked with the other voluntary organisations via the local Council for Voluntary Service or some other 'umbrella' organisation.

Nevertheless, only 70% of the available places are filled, there are problems of staff motivation and morale, substantial use of agency staff and the service is beginning to deteriorate to the point where the intuitive, initial judgement is made that it may be necessary to decommission the service. The 14 dimensions can be plotted as shown in Figure 5.5.

The level of staff expertise in such a service is likely to be high, requiring qualified nursing staff and care staff qualified at least to NVQ level 2 – hence dimension 1 is plotted well above the centre-line (see 1 in Figure 5.5). The level of media interest is likely to be very high because of the direct involvement of some of the parents and carers with the local media (see 2 in Figure 5.5). If the local media do get involved and bearing in mind that some of the management committee are politically active on the local council, this dimension is similarly plotted very high (see 3 in Figure 5.5). There are in total, including support staff, 14 people employed and if there is no redeployment possible there is a high possibility of redundancies (see 4 in Figure 5.5). The resources employed are considerable, involving purpose-built accommodation on prime residential land with substantial modern equipment, so this dimension is also plotted high (see 5 in Figure 5.5). There is a mandatory statutory requirement to provide appropriate care for this particular user group so again this dimension is plotted high on the matrix (see 6 in Figure 5.5). The provider also has a high level of connective and political

Figure 5.5: Practical example II

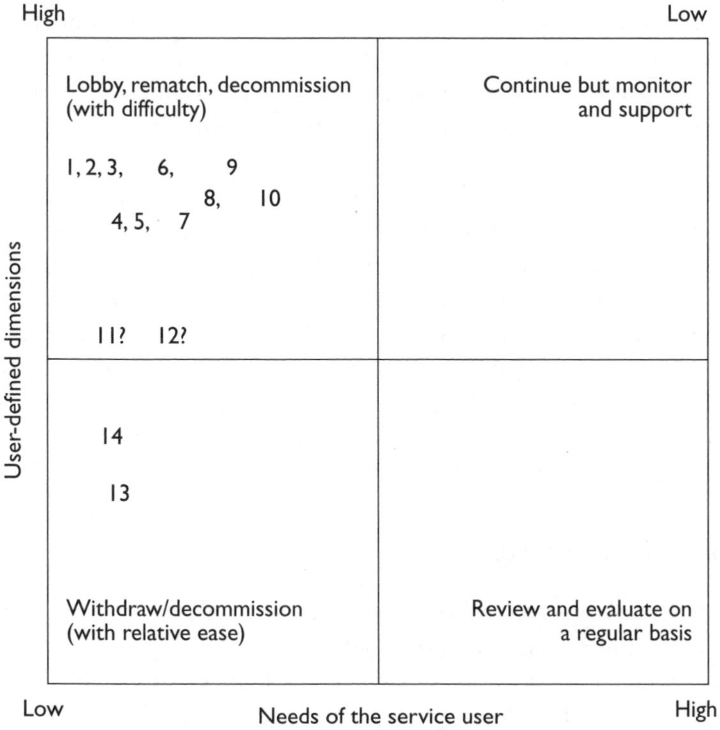

influence, by virtue not only of the involvement of local politicians, but also of the dedicated GP – so again this dimension is plotted high (see 7 in Figure 5.5). It is believed that this provider and others involved in the 'umbrella' organisation have the potential to 'cartel' the commissioner on prices for placements if they so desire. So yet again this dimension is plotted high on the matrix (see 8 in Figure 5.5). At £800 per week for each placement, the financial burden on the commissioner on an annual basis is approximately £42,000 per placement and, assuming 11 placements equate to not far short of half a million pounds per year, this implies a high level of financial expenditure (see 9 in Figure 5.5). If the service is decommissioned it will have severe 'knock-on' effects on other agencies as the provider will then become 'non-viable' and the places commissioned by other agencies will also be lost (see 10 in Figure 5.5). The level of concern by service users and similarly parents or carers is less certain. If they are beginning to notice deterioration in service quality then they may be ambivalent about whether the service is decommissioned, providing, of course, that something better is put in place – so dimensions 11 and 12 are plotted, initially, at the mid-point so as to reflect this uncertainty (see 11 and 12 in Figure 5.5). More consultation will be necessary to make a more precise judgement on these two dimensions so as to determine whether such concern might be positive in that it assists decommissioning, or negative in that it makes it more problematic (see Task 3 and Figure 5.6). The level of monopoly, on the other hand, might be quite low as there may well be other providers or substitute means, such as the provision of extra-care sheltered housing, which will meet the needs of the service users; but remember that 'markets' for social care and health services are sometimes quite tiny: there may be ample provision across the jurisdiction of the commissioning authority but a monopoly at a locality level (see 13 in Figure 5.5). In the latter case, accessibility of the service to its principal users might be quite low, hence dimension 14 is plotted in the lower half of the matrix (see 14 in Figure 5.5).

It is clear from this analysis that as 12 of the dimensions used are in the upper left-hand quadrant then decommissioning this service is going to be exceptionally problematic, yet there may be equally, exceptionally important justifications for so doing. The general implication, however, is that for services that predominately plot in this quadrant, further analysis and work utilising a derivative of Kaplan and Norton's (2004) concept of a 'strategy map' (see below for further discussion) is imperative if a rigorous and robust report that will withstand political scrutiny and legal challenge (and thereby protect the analyst and their authority from acting 'ultra vires' or being shown to have failed to follow a due and proper process) is necessary.

Task 2: Score the dimensions

As with all two-dimensional matrices, the dimensions of the MMDM are measured principally by the simple two-point scale (high-low) as used in the worked examples – which provides four cells. Depending on circumstances, however, it is perfectly feasible for users to adopt a true continuous scale for both axes (thereby providing a more fine-grained measurement of the issues under consideration). In practice, one cannot imagine many situations where a scale of more than 10 points would give any advantage, for to do so would suggest that the issues are amenable to precise measurement whereas manifestly they are not. A 10-point scale, however, is sometimes useful, especially when the plots from Task 1 are evenly spread above and below the centre-line. For example, if one has seven plots in the upper-left quadrant and seven in the lower-left quadrant, some calculation of the scores (six to 10) above the line and (one to five) below the line would add a little extra precision to the analysis. For example, if four of the seven plots above the line scored nine and 10, then this alone would outweigh seven plots below the line and infer that a high resistance to service change will be experienced.

Task 3: Direction of impact of the dimension – negative or positive

Occasionally, where there are a high number of plots above the line or those that are above the line score highly (that is, 8 to 10), then further thought will be required as to whether these particular dimensions are negative (-v) in the sense that they suggest difficulty in decommissioning the service, or positive (+v) in the sense that these dimensions or forces will assist the commissioner in making the case for decommissioning the service. For example, as mentioned earlier, if a service is known over a period of time by the stakeholders involved in it to be under-performing, then a high level of media interest, or a high level of elected member concern, might assist the task of decommissioning the service.

The quadrants

It has become clear through use of the MMDM that the quadrants or cells generated can be given general labels that apply in a wide variety of circumstances. These are withdraw/decommission (with relative ease); lobby, rematch, decommission (with difficulty); continue, but monitor and support; and review and evaluate on a regular basis. They have been thus labelled so as to place political, cultural and social context at the centre of the analysis. This is critical. Public sector organisations are not free to act in ways that their private sector (or even voluntary sector) counterparts can, for all the actions of public sector organisations are subject – to a greater or less degree – to partisan political control or influence and therefore much of what they do is restricted in ways unlike those of other sectors. Accordingly, the labels for the quadrants do not identify strictly 'market-oriented' decisions, but instead identify *actions of engagement with the political, cultural and social process itself.*

As has been revealed, the MMDM provides a robust but relatively simple-to-use intellectual tool for making an initial assessment of the situation. If the analysis reveals that a significant level of difficulty will be experienced in decommissioning a particular service then it implies that there will be a consequent need to undertake further analysis using a derivative of Kaplan and Norton's (2004) concept of a 'strategy map'.

Strategy maps

The aim of a strategy map is to identify and explore the critical components of a strategic decision in a way that reduces the possibility of a flawed decision being made. Applied to the strategic decision to decommission a service it:

- identifies the determinants of the need to decommission a service;
- postulates the principal perspectives that will bear on the decision and need to be taken into account;
- surfaces the critical questions that need to be asked and answered or, at least, responded to;
- provides a framework for a report that recommends the decommissioning of a service that is intellectually and politically as robust as possible.

In Figure 5.6, the determinants of the need to decommission are placed at the centre and the six principal perspectives that will bear on and influence the decision are placed around them.

Figure 5.6: Decommissioning a service

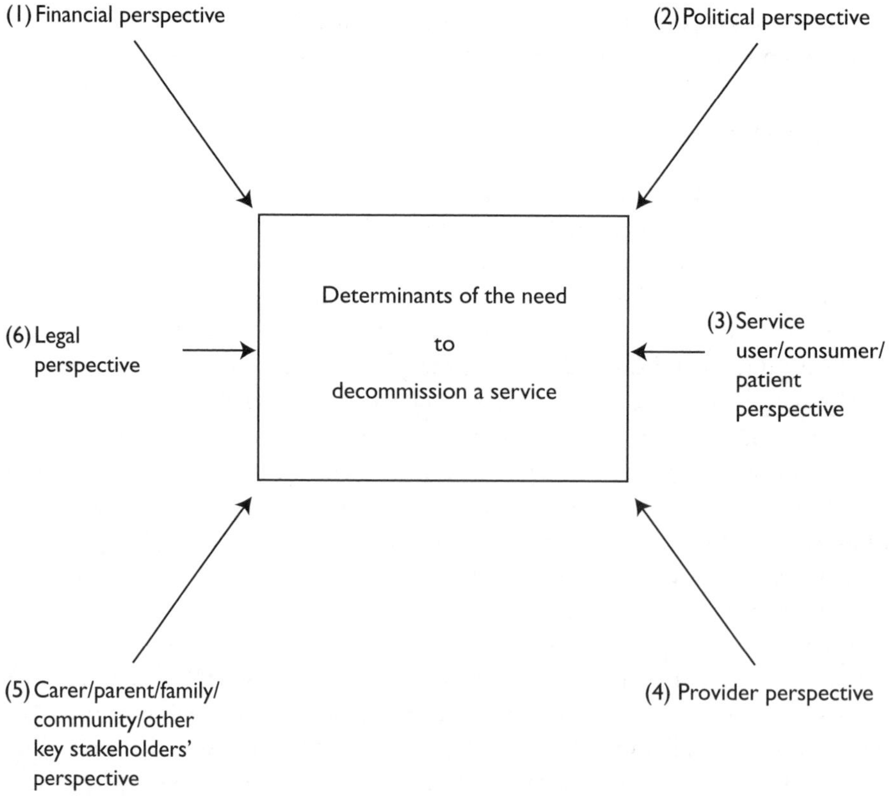

(1) Financial perspective

(2) Political perspective

Determinants of the need
to
decommission a service

(6) Legal perspective

(3) Service user/consumer/ patient perspective

(5) Carer/parent/family/ community/other key stakeholders' perspective

(4) Provider perspective

Determinants of the need to decommission a service

Using the definition of a quality service discussed earlier (that, in essence, it is essentially about getting the best possible *match* between the service provided or procured and the *needs* of the service user and other key stakeholders so that the primary objectives or outcomes desired by or for the service user are achieved), then clearly the first reason to decommission a service is that the service currently provided is ill-matched with the needs of the service user and that it is desirable to achieve a better match.

The second determinant might be to make 'efficiency savings'. The commissioner has been instructed by a higher authority to make, for example, 5% efficiency savings in the cost of provision for a particular service user group. If no cost reduction can be negotiated with the provider, then this may mean the decommissioning of the service, because it does not have the priority accorded to other services and it is the only way of achieving the 5% efficiency savings required.

The third reason for decommissioning a service may be that by so doing it will release resources for more effective use in another service or in another locality within the jurisdiction of the organisation. A fourth determinant might be to relieve pressure on budgets. For example, the service may be, say, £1 million over budget; accordingly, budget reductions are ordered by a higher authority and it is only by decommissioning services that this reduction can be achieved. Increasingly, many public service organisations over the next few years will be required to make budget reductions to reduce the fiscal deficit in the economy and therefore this may become the overriding reason for the decommissioning of services.

A fifth reason may be to ensure that the actual services provided or procured are better matched with the strategic priorities and commissioning action plans of the organisation concerned. It may be found, for example, that some services once deemed necessary are no longer in kilter with changing political or policy priorities and therefore need to be decommissioned. A sixth reason for decommissioning might be that the service has been in receipt of significant adverse comment or publicity from a number of quarters, for a variety of reasons and over a substantial period of time. Although efforts have been made to address such concerns, no improvement has been made and in consequence it is decided to terminate the service, with or without a replacement service being provided.

A seventh reason might be that alternative or substitute provision is now available and, to enable such new provision to grow and flourish, some existing services will need termination. The eighth reason might legitimately be to cope with declining demand for the service. When it was originally provided there was substantial demand and it was viewed as a high-priority service, but due to a change in demography or needs it is now serving only a tiny proportion of service users and therefore it is no longer sufficiently viable in a period of economic dislocation and financial constraint to justify its continued provision.

The ninth determinant of the need to decommission might be that alternative provision to meet the needs of the service user group in question is now available and the existing service has become, to a significant degree, redundant or obsolete and the appropriate response is therefore to decommission it. The tenth determinant – although not perhaps the final determinant, for while this list probably covers the principal reasons, in certain unique situations there may be others of relevance – might be to ensure more equitable treatment of the totality of potential service recipients within the jurisdiction and remit of the public agency concerned. For example, it may be found that a certain group of potential service recipients are currently effectively disenfranchised from any form of provision to meet their needs and yet they manifestly may have needs that justifiably should be met. It may only be that by decommissioning certain existing services, perhaps low-priority ones, that resources can be provided to meet such identified needs.

In practice, there will be usually not one, but a number of related reasons for decommissioning a service; they should be identified and their evidence base fully explored and articulated if a robust case is to be made for recommending a decision to decommission.

Conclusions and next steps: the six perspectives

In coming to a decision to recommend the decommissioning of an especially problematic service (that is, one where many powerful forces are supporting the status quo), six perspectives on the potential decision need to be taken into account. Each of these perspectives generates a number of questions that need exploring and effective responses found if the recommendation to decommission is going to achieve support from relevant interested parties.

The financial perspective

1. The first question assumes that the decommissioning will release resources to be spent on another service or in another locality; therefore, the question becomes: 'Does this release of resources provide a way of accessing other funding streams from other agencies that might enhance the ability to provide a better service for the potential users?'
2. Another important question from the financial perspective might be: 'Would this service be more appropriately funded by a different department, section or agency, which would enhance its viability to the service user and become a more mainstream part of the budget and activities of the new funder?'
3. The third question is: 'What are the likely transaction costs involved in undertaking the decommissioning in question?' By transaction costs we mean largely the staff costs and associated resources necessary to successfully accomplish the task. If it is to be a protracted and difficult exercise, the transaction costs compared with the possible savings or other benefits to be achieved might be minimal and may not therefore be worth the effort involved.

4. Similarly: 'What overheads are attributed to this service and will the commissioning authority still have to bear them, or part of them, if the service is decommissioned?' For example, if Transfer of Undertakings (Protection of Employment) Regulations (TUPE) apply to the staff involved in the service, then depending on the contractual basis under which the service is performed, the redundancy costs and employer-side contribution to the pension funds of such employees may still be borne by the commissioning authority. This feature will presumably have been considered when the service was originally provided or a contract entered into.

5. The fifth question is: 'What percentage of the total spend on the service user group in question will be represented by the decommissioning of a particular service?' Is it, for example, 5% or 70% of the total spending? In the latter case, issues of equity might arise and resources released must necessarily be re-applied to a replacement or substitute service.

6. The sixth question is related, in part, to question (4): 'If redundancies are inevitable, there being no redeployment opportunities available, who will bear them and what likely effects will such redundancies have on the commissioning authority?' If it were a large-scale decommissioning exercise then in a local authority setting it might have significant adverse implications for what might be a key political objective of the local authority (such as its anti-poverty strategy). This again reflects the unique position of public sector organisations, local authorities in particular, in that their concerns are necessarily much wider than those of a private sector, market-oriented organisation.

7. The next question is: 'Will the commissioning authority be involved in any other financial costs arising from the retention or disposal of assets, including intellectual property rights?' For example, it may have been the case that when the service was first provided or the contract created the commissioning authority, in an attempt to assure suitable provision and encourage the provider, took a 30-year lease on a building so as to enable the provider to deliver the service from a particularly favourable location. If after, shall we say, five years a decision, for whatever reason, is made to decommission the service, what is the authority to do with the remaining 25 years of the lease?

8. The answers to the earlier questions will assist in responding to the final question, namely: 'How much money will the commissioning authority save from the decision to decommission the service under review?'

In certain circumstances there may be additional questions to be asked but those outlined above represent the most important ones and will most certainly influence the final decision.

The political perspective

Elected members, other representatives of higher authority, senior managers and other interested parties are all likely to have key regard to the following questions, and the responses to them will influence the level of support that the recommendation to decommission receives:

1. Would the decommissioning, if carried through, promise benefits to the organisation and to those whom it serves? If so:
   i. What are those benefits?
   ii. How do they meet the objectives we are trying to achieve?
   iii. How will they be distributed across the jurisdiction of the organisation in question?
   iv. To whom will they accrue?
   v. When will they accrue?
2. What disadvantages might flow from the decommissioning of the service?
   i. Who would experience them?
   ii. What, if any, remedies would correct them?
   iii. Are the skills and resources for correcting them likely to be available when the disadvantages begin to accrue?
3. What demands will the implementation of this decommissioning make on resources of skilled staff and other resources? Are these resources available?
4. Is there a cheaper, or simpler, way of achieving the suggested decommissioning or at least part of it, and if so:
   i. What would it be?
   ii. What proportion of the total objective would have to be sacrificed if it were adopted?
5. What skills, if any, might be rendered obsolete by the implementation of the decommissioning and what problems would the obsolescence of these skills create for the people who have them?
6. Is the decommissioning one that other similar organisations may have implemented or has it been started and stopped in other organisations? If so, what experience is available from them that might assist with the evaluation of the current proposal?
7. If the decommissioning is *not* implemented, what disadvantages and penalties might accrue to the organisation, the service users or other key stakeholders? Are there any alternative ideas that ought to be considered?
8. If the decommissioning is implemented, what other work in the form of supporting systems should be set in hand simultaneously to:
   i. cope with the consequences of it; or
   ii. prepare for the next stage, and if there is a next stage:
   iii. what would the next stage be?
9. If an initial decision is made to proceed, how long will the option to stop remain open and how reversible will the decision be at progressive stages beyond that?

(This is a crucially important question if it is a large-scale decommissioning exercise that involves substantial assets and resources and is likely to concern many interested parties.)

10. What adverse reactions are likely to arise from affected parties? What actions should be taken to mitigate them? (Amended from Puffitt et al, 1992 and Puffitt, 1993)

Service user/consumer/patient perspective

1. How satisfied is the service user with the current service?
2. What level of complaint or adverse criticism has been received about the service?
3. What level and type of disruption will the service user suffer if the service is changed?
4. Will the service user, if they pay or part-pay for the service, be involved in more or less cost?
5. What is the likely willingness of the service user to bear the changes implied?
6. What effect will it have on the core benefits they receive from the service (for example, safety, security, well-being, timeliness, independence, dignity, confidentiality and responsiveness)?
7. How long will it take for a new service to 'bed down' if one is to be provided?
8. What short-term additional support might the service user need in order to accommodate to the change?
9. Are the resources available to provide any additional support if needed?
10. Is there a need for change in referral processes?
11. What connective or political power does the service user possess that might hinder or help the decommissioning process?

The provider perspective

This perspective is especially important if it is a small-scale provider, irrespective of what sector it is based in, and/or if the commissioning authority wishes it to continue providing other services for the same group, a different service user group or a different locality:

1. What will be the effects of loss of funding for the provider?
2. What are the scale effects (for example, will it remove, say, 80% of the service it provides, thereby rendering it completely non-viable, or a more modest proportion, which will not threaten its continued existence)?
3. What will be the effects on other services, if any, that the provider is involved in?
4. What will be the effects on working relationships between the provider and the commissioning authority?
5. Will there be any redeployment or redundancy issues for the provider?

6. Will the provider need assistance with the realignment of resources? (This again is an important question if the commissioning authority requires its continued existence.)
7. Will the provider need assistance with finding replacement funding?
8. Will the provider need assistance with publicity/promotion issues (for example, whenever a service is decommissioned there is a tendency among the general public to assume that it is because of inadequate performance, with the negative connotations that flow from this, whereas the real reason may be merely declining demand)?
9. What will be the effects on the market of provision? Does it alter the balance of power such that the commissioning authority is disadvantaged?
10. What might be the effects on other providers?

Carer/parent/family/community/other stakeholders' perspective

1. How satisfied are the other stakeholders with the current service?
2. What level of complaint or adverse criticism has been received from them about the current service?
3. What level and type of disruption will the stakeholders suffer if the service is changed?
4. Will the stakeholders be involved in more or less cost?
5. What is the willingness of the stakeholders to bear the change?
6. What effect will it have on the core benefits that the stakeholders receive from the service (for example, respite, dependability, resilience and support)?
7. How long will it take for a new service to 'bed down' if one is to be provided?
8. What short-term additional support might the stakeholders need in order to accommodate the change?
9. Are there resources available to provide any additional support if needed?
10. Will the stakeholders be affected by any necessary change in referral processes?
11. What connective or political power do the stakeholders possess that might hinder or help the decommissioning process?

The legal perspective

Any manager formulating a report that recommends a decision to decommission a service will require detailed advice from legally qualified colleagues. At the very least, the following questions will need addressing:

1. At what level should consultation on the proposals take place? It may require consultation at three different levels: (i) a strategic level; (ii) an operational/ tactical level; and (iii) an individual/human rights level. For example, if the commissioning authority were to reduce, say, its grant budget for voluntary organisations by 20% in a particular year, it will first need to consult with the 'umbrella' organisation representing voluntary organisations in the area

(probably the local Council for Voluntary Service) as to the overall effects that such a reduction might have. Moreover, if that 20% reduction were to have a disproportionate effect on a particular category of voluntary organisation, say those providing services for partially sighted people, then it will need to consult directly with that category of voluntary organisation (that is to say, at the operational/tactical level). Third, it will need to consult directly with those individual service users who might lose service if the grant cut is implemented. All three levels of consultation will need to have proper regard to the following:

- The duration of the consultation period must be considered.
- It must be undertaken at a formative stage of the decision-making process.
- It must provide adequate time for effective responses to be made.
- It must show that the views expressed have been taken into account.
- There must be a specific process for giving feedback to the consultees.
- There must be full compliance with any consultation protocols that are in place.

2. Are the human rights of any service user or stakeholder disadvantaged by the proposal to decommission?
3. In what circumstances will TUPE and associated statutory instruments apply?
4. Does the proposal affect the pension rights of employees of the provider?
5. Is the proposal likely to create a two-tier workforce whereby some employees are disadvantaged?
6. Are there internal protocols or contract documents in place that provide for service change?
7. Will there be termination payments, damages and other kinds of end-of-service issues to be taken into account?
8. At the termination of the service, is it clear who owns land, property, intellectual property and other assets and resources, including confidential information and records?
9. Has a rigorous analysis of the legal risks and the management of those risks been undertaken by the commissioning authority with a view to deterring or at least being able to withstand legal challenge by way of civil litigation, judicial review of the processes employed, or by the organisation being held as acting outside of, or beyond, its powers

In total, the questions generated from these six perspectives might be regarded as somewhat onerous, but if safe and proper decisions are to be made, especially for the more problematic decommissioning exercises where powerful forces are supporting the status quo, then to ask and formulate answers to these questions is fundamentally important. However, public sector decisions can never be completely optimising in a strictly commercial sense and, while careful analysis might suggest that a service be decommissioned, so powerful might be the forces supporting the status quo that the manager concerned might be powerless by economic logic alone to effect the necessary changes. If this is the case then the implication is that they must temporarily disengage themselves from the potential recommendation to decommission and await a change in political, cultural or social forces that might lead to a more propitious set of circumstances and a more positive environment in which to effect the necessary changes. This is the reality of life in a public sector setting.

Further reading

This is an area about which little is written – and the ideas and frameworks in this chapter have been specifically designed to support public service commissioners in this neglected area. However, additional sources include:

- Donaldson, C., Bate, A., Mitton, C., Dionne, F. and Ruta, D. (2010) 'Rational disinvestment', QJM, vol 103, no 10, pp 801-7.
- Elshaug, A. G., Moss, J. R., Littlejohns, P., Karnon, J., Merlin, T. L. and Hiller, J. E. (2009) 'Identifying existing health care services that do not provide value for money', *Medical Journal of Australia*, vol 190, pp 269-73.
- Robinson, S., Dickinson, H., Freeman, T. and Williams, I. (2011) 'Disinvestment in health: the challenges facing general practitioner (GP) commissioners', *Public Money and Management*, vol 31, no 2, pp 145-48.
- Williams, I., Robinson, S. and Dickinson, H. (2011) *Rationing in health care: the theory and practice of priority setting*, Bristol: The Policy Press.

Useful websites

- Commissioning Options Appraisal Tool (2009): www.dcsf.gov.uk/ everychildmatters/strategy/managersandleaders/planningandcommissioning/ about/aboutprocess/
- The National Institute for Health and Clinical Excellence (NICE) has compiled a 'do not do' database of obsolete healthcare practices: www.nice.org.uk/ usingguidance/donotdorecommendations/detail.jsp
- The National Institute for Innovation and Improvement has designed a toolkit for those charged with making 'tough choices' over the allocation of scarce resources: www.institute.nhs.uk/world_class_commissioning/tackling_tough_ choices/tackling_tough_choices_creating_public_value_homepage.html

Reflective exercises

This is a very practical chapter already, but using the MMDM set out above, analyse a local service that has been identified as under-performing/not delivering best value for money to explore whether you think that it should be considered for decommissioning, what reaction this might produce and how you would manage the process.

If you decide to recommend decommissioning, apply the six perspectives discussed above to consider the implications that your decision may have and plan potential responses.

References

Department of the Environment, Transport and the Regions (1999) Circular 10/99 'Implementing Best Value', London: DETR

Kaplan, R. S. and Norton, D. P. (2004) *Strategy maps*, Boston, MA: Harvard Business School Press.

Puffitt, R. G. (1993) *Business planning and marketing: a guide for the local government cost centre manager*, London: Longman.

Puffitt, R. G., Stoten, B. and Winkley, D. (1992) *Business planning for schools*, London: Longman.

Prince, L. P. and Puffitt, R. G. (2001) 'The Maslin Multi-Dimensional Matrix: a new tool to aid strategic decision making in the public sector', in G. Johnson and K. Scholes (eds) *Exploring public sector strategy*, London: Prentice Hall and *The Financial Times*, pp 143-64.

SIX

Commissioning for service resilience

Ray Puffitt

Summary

This chapter explores:

• key financial challenges and the need to consider the resilience of service providers;
• a practical framework for assessing resilience/vulnerability;
• a worked example of the framework in action;
• the importance of service continuity planning.

In the preceding chapter, the underpinnings, the rationale and the means of using the Maslin Multi-Dimensional Matrix (MMDM) as an aid to strategic decision making were outlined and the matrix was applied to the decommissioning of services. In this chapter, it is applied to a different topic, namely 'commissioning for service resilience in the face of economic dislocation and financial restraint'. Over the next few years, all providers of services – whether provided in-house, by the market or by the voluntary and community sector – will be faced with the aftermath of the near collapse of the global financial economy. This has resulted in an exceptionally volatile environment. Some providers will cope with the changes, while others will experience difficulty, sometimes leading to the possibility of significant service deterioration or even provider collapse. This poses the question: Why it is that some providers fail to adapt to a changing environment? In particular, what dimensions or factors contribute to this lack of resilience and inability to manage change?

In broad terms, the reasons why organisations fail to adapt to a changing environment can be grouped as follows:

1. Insufficient information about and, analysis of, all the factors affecting their ability to achieve objectives and outcomes, including the constraints and restraints. There is a fundamental difference between constraints and restraints, which is especially important for public service organisations. The definition of 'constraints' is: 'incidents, events, or contingencies completely beyond the influence or control of the organisation which confine or compel the actions or decisions available to the organisation' (Puffitt, 1993, p 95). The only way

an organisation can deal with constraints is to identify them and then avoid taking action that compounds their adverse effects.

Naturally, constraints bear upon both private and public sector organisations, but in public sector organisations it is the definition of 'restraints' that is of particular importance. Restraints are 'those actions or decisions which an organisation takes on moral or political grounds whether or not such actions or decisions improve the ability to reach primary objectives or outcomes' (Puffitt, 1993, p 95). By and large, private sector organisations restrict the number of self-imposed restraints they put upon themselves in pursuit of their objectives, whereas public sector organisations, local authorities in particular, have a tendency to almost maximise them. In a way, this is to be expected because the role of the latter is to balance competing values, objectives and interests. This creates no problem if they have surfaced what adverse results such self-imposed restraints might have on their ability to achieve their primary objective and are prepared to accept the consequences.

However, it does become a problem if they have failed to undertake this exploration, for then it becomes more difficult to achieve primary objectives. For example, the decision might be made to convert the entirety of the organisation's vehicle fleet to liquid petroleum gas (LPG) for no other reason than it is deemed an interesting thing to do. There is no mandatory requirement for this to happen yet this self-imposed restraint may, at least for a period of time, restrict the ability of the transport fleet to meet its primary objective of transporting people, equipment, substances and so on about the area with a high degree of economy, efficiency and effectiveness. Some vehicles will be off-the-road having their engines converted to run on LPG, while others, which unconverted may have had a future useful life, will have to be disposed of and new vehicles purchased. This is often a feature of public sector service specifications where large numbers of what are no more than 'restraints' are inserted into the specification at the expense of economy, efficiency and effectiveness in the achievement of the primary objectives and outcomes of the service. We return to this issue of self-imposed restraints when discussing service continuity plans in the later stages of this chapter.

2. Inadequate leadership capability is another organisational problem that may result in a lack of directional clarity, whereby inadequate distinction is made between what are the primary objectives of the service, as compared with what are only critical or non-critical secondary objectives (that is to say, they are merely the means by which primary objectives are achieved) (Delderfield et al, 1991). That is not to say that they have no importance, but that they should not be pursued with the vigour accorded to primary objectives. They must not become an end in themselves and thereby obscure what is of priority in the delivery of the service. Another aspect of inadequate leadership capability is evidenced by the organisation that is clear about what it really wants to achieve but has insufficient 'managerial grip' to make it actually happen.

3. Ineffective structural capability may also sometimes be a problem in two ways: (a) the organisation is the wrong structural shape – what is required may be a highly decentralised organisation whereas in practice the organisation has a tendency to be centrally driven and directed, which makes it difficult to achieve its objectives or vice versa; (b) ineffectual operating systems and processes may be another manifestation of an organisation that is predisposed to fail to adapt to a changing environment. All the management literatures have emphasised the importance of effective systems and processes to support the organisation in pursuit of its aims.

4. Inappropriate cultural capability, which may be manifested in one or more of three particular ways:
   • misaligned values, that is to say, out of kilter with the values of the commissioning authority – this will at best result in strained working relationships between provider and commissioner and at worst an inability to achieve the objectives desired by the commissioner;
   • the organisation that is bedevilled by 'historical habits' – preferred ways of doing things, or particular organisational objectives, that inhibit the achievement of what is required by the commissioning authority;
   • a distinct lack of congruence between the objectives of the provider and prevalent national or local policy imperatives.
   In essence, the objectives of the provider are out of step with changing norms, values and the intentions behind new policy initiatives.

This broad grouping of the reasons why organisations fail to adapt to a changing environment is later in this chapter broken down to approximately 45 specific issues that form the dimensions or factors for the y-axis when using the MMDM to identify the vulnerability of a provider to a changing environment (see the previous chapter for further details of the MMDM approach).

Changing contextual factors

Although the detail is beyond the remit of this chapter, the principal contextual factors that are likely to affect the ability of providers to continue to ensure effective service delivery are set out in Figure 6.1.

Of course, many of these factors are in play at a time of increasing demand for public services. This is creating a situation where public service commissioning staff across the United Kingdom are faced with the possibility of service deterioration – and in some instances provider collapse – as the market of provision attempts to cope with a rapidly changing environment. It becomes essential, therefore, for the commissioner to identify those services and providers that are the least resilient and therefore the most vulnerable to service deterioration or collapse, with a view to deciding what, if any, support they may need to continue to deliver an acceptable service. Using the MMDM approach from the previous chapter will enable the user to plot on the matrix all the dimensions or factors that are likely to lead to lack of resilience and hence vulnerability to changing market conditions. Figure 6.1 illustrates how the dimensions as factors are interrelated with the changing context.

Figure 6.1: Changing contextual factors

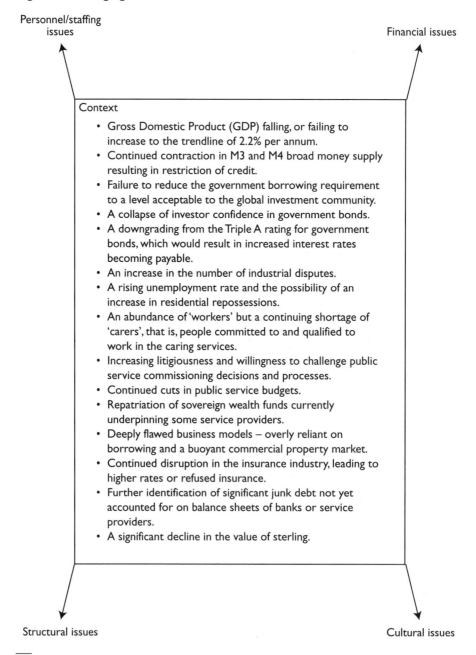

Personnel/staffing issues

Financial issues

Context
- Gross Domestic Product (GDP) falling, or failing to increase to the trendline of 2.2% per annum.
- Continued contraction in M3 and M4 broad money supply resulting in restriction of credit.
- Failure to reduce the government borrowing requirement to a level acceptable to the global investment community.
- A collapse of investor confidence in government bonds.
- A downgrading from the Triple A rating for government bonds, which would result in increased interest rates becoming payable.
- An increase in the number of industrial disputes.
- A rising unemployment rate and the possibility of an increase in residential repossessions.
- An abundance of 'workers' but a continuing shortage of 'carers', that is, people committed to and qualified to work in the caring services.
- Increasing litigiousness and willingness to challenge public service commissioning decisions and processes.
- Continued cuts in public service budgets.
- Repatriation of sovereign wealth funds currently underpinning some service providers.
- Deeply flawed business models – overly reliant on borrowing and a buoyant commercial property market.
- Continued disruption in the insurance industry, leading to higher rates or refused insurance.
- Further identification of significant junk debt not yet accounted for on balance sheets of banks or service providers.
- A significant decline in the value of sterling.

Structural issues

Cultural issues

Of course, as the contextual factors change, they tend to make the personnel, financial, cultural and structural issues more (or less) problematic. For example, if GDP falls then it is likely to make some of these issues more difficult to deal with and vice versa.

Using the MMDM

As for the preceding chapter, the dimension for the x-axis is again 'need for the service as currently provided', but on this occasion of use the assumption is made that there is a *high* need for the service as currently provided. The service might not in practice be 'gold plated' or even reach the Best Value target area, but nevertheless it is an acceptable service, fit for its purpose and one certainly does not want the service to deteriorate below the current standard nor for the provider to collapse. Accordingly, on this occasion of use we are using the right-hand side of the matrix to identify where there is a *poor* match, as opposed to a *good match*, between the dimensions on the x-axis and the dimensions on the y-axis – for this will indicate which dimensions/factors of the 45 or so explored are leading to vulnerability to service deterioration or provider collapse. In essence, it identifies the linkages between the service provided and the dimensions/factors affecting its resilience and hence vulnerability (see Figure 6.2).

Figure 6.2: The MMDM approach

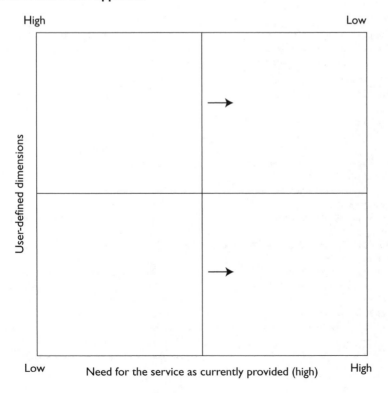

In undertaking the analysis, a simple high/low rating is appropriate where high implies vulnerability. For example, where a service exhibits a high level of staff turnover, or has a high level of borrowing, or manifests a high level of lack of congruence with national imperatives or has a high level of underused capacity and so on, this would clearly indicate a number of weaknesses/problems that would need addressing if the service was not to suffer deterioration or the possibility of collapse.

Box 6.1 presents examples of dimensions that could be used on the y-axis and which, if plotted high, and therefore falling in the top right-hand quadrant of the matrix, would indicate a significant likelihood of service deterioration or collapse when faced with changes in the context. The relative importance of each will vary to some extent with the particular service being analysed.

Box 6.1: Indicators of vulnerability

Personnel/staffing issues	Financial issues
level of 1 Need for high skilled staff	level of 13 Need for land and buildings
level of 2 Need for qualified staff	level of 14 Capital required
level of 3 Inability to recruit requisite staff	level of 15 Buildings
level of 4 Staff turnover	level of 16 Interest payments on borrowings
level of 5 Staff absences	level of 17 Interest rate paid
level of 6 Use of agency staff	level of 18 Probability of breaching banking covenants
level of 7 Problematic staff morale	level of 19 Rent/lease payments
level of 8 Inability to cope with load	level of 20 Insurance required
level of 9 Inadequacy of admin/clerical support	level of 21 Need for liquidity/cash flow
level of 10 Inadequacy of IT support	level of 22 Unavailability of accurate cost data
level of 11 Obsolescent staff skills	level of 23 Inadequacy of surplus/profit
level of 12 Unavailability of in-house training	level of 24 Overheads

Cultural issues	Structural issues
level of 25 Change in values	level of 36 Unavailability/inadequacy of appropriate equipment
level of 26 Change in objectives	level of 37 Inappropriate location (to main users)
level of 27 Change in priorities	level of 38 Unsuitable structural shape eg centralised v. decentralised
level of 28 Lack of congruence with national imperatives	level of 39 Inadequate premises from which to deliver services
level of 29 Lack of congruence with local imperatives	level of 40 Underused capacity/voids
level of 30 Inadequate compliance with statutory rules	level of 41 Threat of new entrants/substitutes
level of 31 Inadequate compliance with local protocols	level of 42 Dependence on suppliers of resources
level of 32 Lack of directional clarity/focus	level of 43 Possibility of decline in demand
level of 33 Historical habits	level of 44 Turbulence in the management/ administrative structure
level of 34 Resistance to change	level of 45 Lack of loyalty of user group
level of 35 Rigidity (wish to change but cannot)	level of 46 Lack of loyalty of political interests
	level of 47 & 48 (Market share) from both the purchaser and the provider perspective

To summarise, plot all 48 dimensions (and other relevant self-generated ones) either high or low on the right-hand side of the matrix using the allotted numbers to do so. This will assist the analyst in: (a) identifying the level of vulnerability of the service; (b) highlighting which are the principal issues leading to that vulnerability; and (c) by implication suggesting what actions may need to be taken to address the weaknesses exposed.

A case study: community equipment

To illustrate the use of the matrix in this way, we take the example of a newly established integrated community equipment store – the principal prescribers being occupational therapists, surgeons, domiciliary nurses, general practitioners (GPs) and social workers. The existing provider won the new contract on the basis of a very keen price, the quality of the pre-existing service and the good relationships already established. But, of course, this is a *new* service, which now provides over 500 different pieces of equipment on loan, funded by a Section 75 agreement between the local authority and the four primary care trusts (PCTs) within its area (soon to be new GP consortia). The local authority holds the budget and budget manages the funds.

The financial arrangement is that the provider purchases, warehouses, delivers, installs, maintains and collects community equipment for daily living, rehabilitation and community use for which they are paid. Sixty per cent of the equipment is recycled for subsequent use, but this itself sometimes creates problems as service users have high expectations and, in consequence, there are often complaints about the equipment being 'second-hand'.

Critical to the success of the service is:

- a good database coupled with effective liaison between the 850 prescribers, service users and the provider so as to ensure prompt return of equipment when no longer needed or to deal with product recalls, thereby reducing the cost of holding surplus or obsolescent equipment in store;
- accurate and comprehensive completion by the 850 prescribers of the requisition forms so as to avoid rejection of the form for lack of data by the provider (with so many prescribers there is a consequent need for ongoing training of prescribers in these requirements);
- a positive, constructive and harmonious relationship between all prescribers and the provider's customer service staff;
- ample fund availability to the provider to enable it to purchase and hold some £300,000 of equipment in store, thereby reducing delays in delivery and being able to grow the service in accordance with Department of Health requirements to increase the number of clients served by 50% in three years;
- the payment of invoices on receipt, with discrepancies dealt with later, so as to maintain the liquidity of the provider;

- the ability of the provider to recruit and retain staff with the competence and commitment to maintain a good service (that is, 95% of deliveries on time) and sound relationships with the prescribers and service users;
- the ability of the provider to develop effective links with its suppliers of equipment (currently just in excess of 1,000);
- the prescribers' knowledge of and familiarity with the catalogue of available equipment and, in particular, their knowledge of up-to-date equipment (as opposed to what may have been in use some 20 years earlier when they qualified) plus the ability to measure and prescribe accurately in both imperial and metric measurements;
- the existence of a suitable database on who is prescribing what equipment and at what cost, so as to ensure that local budgets are effectively managed and overspends curtailed.

Doubts as to the viability of the contract were raised within six months of commencement arising from the financial viability of the provider to cope with the need to purchase, warehouse and transport additional equipment. However, this problem was averted by the parent company, a manufacturer of assistive technology equipment, investing a further £600,000 in its subsidiary. Also, but unbeknown to the purchaser, it was agreed that the contract would be cross-subsidised by the surpluses made on six other contracts, which enjoy much more favourable returns, in the hope that over the five-year life of the contract it would yield a 10% surplus overall.

Until recently the provider has been performing well and meeting its targets but at the expense of considerable staff turnover arising from the work pressures experienced by the driver/technicians and customer service staff. These problems are compounded by difficulties in recruiting and retaining suitable staff, but by extensive cross-zone working (there are 10 delivery zones in the area), this problem is temporarily averted – but with consequent knock-on costs for the staff involved.

To maximise the use of driver/technician time, a system has been introduced at the warehouse of utilising 'order pickers' to load the delivery vehicles before the commencement of the delivery day. However, this solution fails if a driver fails to turn up for work (a frequent occurrence) and then the orders have to be reallocated to other delivery vehicles, thereby putting additional strain on the drivers concerned. Moreover, the customer service staff are regularly in receipt of abusive comments and involved in heated exchanges with some of the prescribers who fail to appreciate the pressure they work under.

From the commissioner's perspective there are overspends on the PCT budgets primarily created by some clinicians insisting on delivery to hospital wards and departments for which they have to pay per delivery as opposed to bulk delivery of a range of equipment to peripheral stores for which there is only one delivery payment made.

Currently, these overspends are allocated according to the financial contributions to the pooled budget paid by the particular PCT, but in future it is intended that the totality of the overspend will be attributed to the overspending PCT. This in itself will add to the tensions articulated at the bi-monthly meeting of the partnership board – at which tensions tend to revolve around the prescribing patterns of each of the different prescribing groups. These tensions are repeated at the monthly equipment review meetings where decisions are made as to what new equipment should be stocked, with each prescribing group arguing for its own preferences.

The service is glued together by the excellent relationship between the local authority's project manager and the manager of the warehouse, but there are doubts as to whether this can continue in the face of the potential difficulties arising from the overall viability of this particular contract. Moreover, the project manager holds the post for only a further 18 months and, given a change in personalities and therefore relationships, the contract could easily fail.

Matters have just come to a head as both the project manager and the warehouse manager have announced their intention to move to other positions. There is no succession planning in place. Furthermore, over the past four weeks, late delivery has increased with on-time delivery slipping to 80%, with consequent complaints from both service users and prescribers. In part, this is due to prescribers specifying urgent delivery (that is, within four hours), with this requirement now rising to 15% of the total requisitions. Moreover, the provider is failing to notify the prescribers of such late delivery within the target of 24 hours. The retrieval rate has also fallen below the target of 55%.

Plotting this service on the matrix using the dimensions derived from the four key perspectives produces roughly the pattern shown on Figure 6.3 and reveals that there are predominantly personnel, financial and some structural issues that need addressing. Although there are a substantial number of issues that plot in the lower right-hand quadrant (which indicates that at the time of evaluation they were not problematic), these may become more significant over time because of the turbulence in the environment. They therefore require reviewing and evaluation on a regular basis.

In practice, it would be worthwhile to list from the top right-hand quadrant a number of the principal issues, in order of perceived priority, so as to focus the analyst's attention on matters that need addressing with relative urgency.

Conclusion: service continuity planning

Obviously, these issues will raise concerns for the commissioner about the ongoing viability of the service, so there is a need to formulate a range of actions by which to mitigate the weaknesses exposed and which will form part of a service continuity plan. Such action might include the following, starting with the simplest:

1. Discussions with the provider about the problems as the commissioner sees them. The provider may be aware only of a limited number of issues that concern them and may not have undertaken such a rigorous analysis as has the

Figure 6.3: Practical example

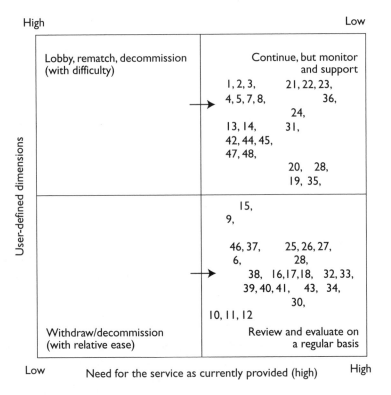

(Right-hand side of the matrix)

	High	Low
	Lobby, rematch, decommission (with difficulty)	Continue, but monitor and support 1, 2, 3, 21, 22, 23, 4, 5, 7, 8, 36, 24, 13, 14, 31, 42, 44, 45, 47, 48, 20, 28, 19, 35,
		15, 9, 46, 37, 25, 26, 27, 6, 28, 38, 16, 17, 18, 32, 33, 39, 40, 41, 43, 34, 30, 10, 11, 12
	Withdraw/decommission (with relative ease)	Review and evaluate on a regular basis

User-defined dimensions

Low   Need for the service as currently provided (high)   High

commissioner. This is a particular problem with smaller providers, irrespective of which sector they are based in. When such issues are raised formally, the provider themselves may be able to address them without further assistance from the commissioner.

2. Support the provider by applying, perhaps only on a short-term basis to overcome a transient difficulty, additional resources by way of:
   • amendment of the payment terms to facilitate their cash flow/liquidity position, which in turn will provide them with greater credibility with their banking facilities via enhanced credit opportunities and more favourable relationships and possible discounts from their suppliers;
   • putting staff into the provider's organisation on a temporary basis to support continued delivery of the service;
   • provide other resources such as property, equipment, training, consultancy and advice.

3. Revisit the service specification with a view to reducing the number of constraints, non-critical secondary objectives and, in particular, the restraints so as to enable the provider to focus their efforts on what is of primary rather than lesser importance.

4. Assist the provider to gain greater control or influence over their sources of supply of resources. For example, if they lack and need certain equipment (for example furniture for use in their facility), it may be possible to use the commissioner's central-purchasing function to supply such equipment at cost. Similarly, if the commissioning authority has its own in-house recruitment agency, or temporary staff agency or training facility, then again it may be able to offer a service at cost to the provider, thereby lessening their dependence on others.
5. Increase the volume of work made available to the provider so that it can spread its overheads either alone or in consortia arrangement with other authorities.
6. If the issues of concern are predominantly financial, then other issues being favourable, it might be helpful to encourage the provider to innovate so as to develop services of greater value to the commissioning authority, for which a larger payment can be made, hence increasing the level of surplus available to the provider and thereby enhancing its viability.
7. If all else fails and where mandatory statutory objectives are involved, then the commissioning authority has to consider the possibility of bringing the service back in-house either alone or with other authorities.

All these actions should take account of procurement law and how other providers might perceive them, for one must maintain a 'level playing field'.

Finally, an intensely sensitive political decision has to be made. Does the commissioning authority by its action try to support providers that are vulnerable to service deterioration or collapse by virtue of changes in economic or financial circumstances or does it stand back, allow them to fail and focus all its efforts on the strongest providers with the proviso that in so doing, they are still able to fulfil their statutory duties. This decision will naturally require sign-off at the very highest level.

Further reading/useful websites

Like Chapter Five, this is an area about which little is written (but which is very topical in the current financial climate) – and the ideas and frameworks in this chapter have been specifically designed to support public service commissioners in this neglected area. However, additional resources include a 2010 government guide entitled *How to: manage the risk of significant disruption to services in an economic downturn* (see http://webarchive.nationalarchives.gov.uk/20100612131212/dcsf. gov.uk/everychildmatters/resources-and-practice/ig00708/)

The Department of Health has published a provider economics impact assessment model to explore how commissioning/decommissioning decisions might impact on provider sustainability: Department of Health and NHS Confederation (2010) *Provider economics impact assessment model*, London: Department of Health, www.dh.gov.uk/en/Publicationsandstatistics/Publications/PublicationsPolicyAndGuidance/DH_122570.

Reflective exercises

This is a very practical chapter already – but using the MMDM set out above, analyse a local case study service to consider its vulnerability/resilience and explore possible steps for boosting its resilience.

References

Delderfield, J., Puffitt, R. G. and Watts, G. (1991) *Business planning in local government*, London: Longman.

Puffitt, R. G. (1993) *Business planning and marketing: a guide for the local government cost central manager*, London: Longman.

Puffitt, R. G., Stoten, B. and Winkley, D. (1992) *Business planning for schools*, London: Longman.

SEVEN

Commissioning for quality and outcomes

Martin Willis and Tony Bovaird

Summary

This chapter explores:
- definitions of quality and outcomes in health and social care;
- an outcome-based commissioning cycle in policy and practice;
- outcomes that matter to service users;
- co-commissioning and co-production.

'Quality' and 'outcomes' are slippery concepts that become even harder to pin down when applied to the practice of health and social care. As such, they have proved to be rich territory for both academic study and policy guidance since the public sector took on board the customer-focused exhortations of the Total Quality Management gurus in the 1980s (Peters and Waterman, 1982; Morgan and Murgatroyd, 1994).

Both children's and adults' social care have seen major investments in academic research aimed at defining and specifying outcomes. The pioneering work on outcomes for children at the Dartington Social Research Unit (Parker et al, 1991) has led to statutory recognition of 'the five outcomes which mattered most to children and young people' in the *Every child matters* Green Paper (HM Treasury, 2003, p 6) and the subsequent Children Act 2004. In adult care, the Social Policy Research Unit (SPRU) has specified an outcomes framework that distinguishes between maintenance, change and process outcomes (Qureshi, 2000) and the government has proposed seven 'clear outcomes for social care' (DH, 2005, p 10). More recently, the new Liberal-Conservative coalition government has also emphasised a more outcomes-based approach to the delivery of public services – although much of the detail is still to emerge at the time of writing.

Inspection evidence supports the contention that achieving an outcome focus in practice has been problematic. Two consecutive annual reports by the former Audit Commission and Social Services Inspectorate Joint Reviews highlighted weaknesses at strategic and frontline practice levels respectively:

> Many of the strategic plans produced by councils do not as yet show how aspirations will be turned into practice, identifying, for example, changes in resource allocation or clear performance targets. Councils need to concentrate on outcome oriented planning rather than on the production of descriptive plans. (Audit Commission and SSI, 1999, p 6)

> It is rare to see the desired outcome of any service in the care plan or written in the case file. For over a decade, social care policy has emphasised the importance of needs-led rather than service-led social care. This appears hard to achieve. What is asked of authorities is that they examine the outcomes that the services achieve for the service user. (Audit Commission and SSI, 2000, p 5)

Over the subsequent 10 years, progress towards establishing a firm understanding of outcomes continued to be slow. For example, Lord Laming's inquiry into the death of Victoria Climbié concluded that '[t]his inquiry saw too many examples of those in senior positions attempting to justify their work in terms of bureaucratic activity, rather than outcomes for people' (DH, 2003, p 6). One of the recommendations of this inquiry was that strategic partnerships should be established at local authority level to coordinate the planning and delivery of children's services. However, the Audit Commission (2008a, p 4) found that '[f]ive years after the Laming enquiry, there is little evidence that children's trusts have improved outcomes for children'.

The story is repeated in research with adult social care users and older people. Shaping Our Lives (2003) worked with two black mental health service users' organisations, a third run by black disabled people and another by older people to explore their experiences of social care services. One stark finding was that '[u]sers felt that services continued to show a lack of respect. The value of their own outcomes was not acknowledged nor valued' (2003, p 1). And at strategic level, the Audit Commission (2008b, p 32) concluded that one of four reasons why the government's *Opportunity age* policy (HM Government, 2005) had 'had little impact on the performance of councils' was because 'the outcomes that councils need to deliver are not defined'.

Early initiatives to promote the concept of 'commissioning' were primarily concerned with the structural coordination of health and social care and financial efficiency and lacked a specific emphasis on quality and outcomes. Knapp et al (1992) argued that the-then Conservative government's promotion of joint commissioning would enable greater consistency in eligibility criteria and foster cooperation rather than passing the buck between health and social care. The arrival of the New Labour government in 1997 resulted in little change in this preoccupation with procedure and structure as witnessed in the Health Act 1999 provisions, which 'created a duty of partnership but also significantly extended the ability of local authorities and the NHS to pool budgets for specific groups of services, delegate commissioning to a "local" organisation and create single provider organisations' (Means et al, 2003, p 113; Clarke and Glendinning, 2002). Similarly, the general practitioner (GP) practice-based commissioning policy was announced in 2004 with only two references to quality and none to outcomes, in contrast to over 50 references to budgets (DH, 2004). Even the widely cited Institute of Public Care's framework, with its emphasis on the links between commissioning, purchasing and contracting, makes no explicit reference to quality or outcomes (Richardson, 2006).

More recent years have seen the promulgation of the notion that quality and outcomes are both integral to, and positively promoted by, health and social care commissioning. But before that is explored, it is necessary to unravel the complexity of what is meant by quality and outcomes in health and social care.

Quality and outcomes

Bovaird and Löffler (2003, 2009) have identified five different concepts of 'quality' during its evolution in public management theory:

- quality as *'conformance to specification'* (a meaning derived from an engineering perspective and from the 'contract culture');
- quality as *'fitness for purpose'* (or 'meeting organisational objectives', essentially derived from a systems perspective);
- quality as *'aligning inputs, process, outputs and outcomes'* (derived from the strategic management perspective);
- quality as *'meeting customer expectations'* (or 'exceeding customer expectation', derived from consumer psychology);
- quality as *'passionate emotional involvement'* – quality as that 'which lies beyond language and number' (the social psychology approach).

This typology has interesting connections with one of the earliest attempts to work with public sector staff and consumer groups in Newcastle and Cambridgeshire to 'encourage local authorities to become more "consumer responsive" in the way they plan and deliver services and to strive for true value for money' (NCC, 1986, p ii). The National Consumer Council (NCC) framework started with five key criteria for service evaluation, expressed in straightforward language:

- *'what is it supposed to do?'* (specifications);
- *'does it do what it is supposed to do?'* (fitness for purpose)
- *'does it do what it is not supposed to do?'* (not fit for purpose);
- *'what does it cost?'* (aligning inputs and outputs efficiently);
- *'what is it like to use?'* (the customer's experience).

Thus, already, quality is being defined in terms of not just the quality of life 'technical' dimensions of a service but also the quality of service experience – 'non-technical' dimensions of the interaction between the consumer, the service and the people delivering the service (Donabedian, 1980, 1982, 1985; Skelcher, 1992; Gaster, 1995; Gaster and Squires, 2003; Forder et al, 2007). Interestingly, the outcomes defined for children (HM Treasury, 2003) focus exclusively on quality dimensions (being healthy; staying safe; enjoying and achieving; making a positive contribution; and economic well-being) whereas the adult outcomes (DH, 2005) include quality of service experience aspects (choice and control; freedom from discrimination or harassment; and personal dignity). More recently, Lord Darzi (2008, p 11), in his major review of the National Health Service (NHS), echoed this duality of what a service is designed to achieve and how it is experienced in stating that 'high quality care should be as safe and effective as possible, with patients treated with compassion, dignity and respect'.

How, then, does this relate to the concept of 'outcomes'? Are the terms 'quality' and 'outcomes' interchangeable as ways of expressing a measurement of the value of a public service? Smith (1996, p 1), in a pioneering text, started from a broad, but 'vague' dictionary definition of an outcome as 'the issue: consequence: result' and then sought to make this more specific. Davies et al, in their exploration of evidence-based public policy and practice, considered the personal subjectivity of determining appropriate outcome measures and argued that '[o]ne of the major challenges of establishing best evidence is doing so in terms of outcomes that are meaningful and relevant to the people who are affected by the interventions concerned' (Davies et al, 2000, p 298).

The struggle to achieve both precision and relevance is evident in the search to define social care and health outcomes. For example, the SPRU research programme on outcomes in social care interpreted 'outcome' 'as the impact or effect on the lives of service users or carers and the emphasis of the programme is on non-clinical, or social care, outcomes rather than health care outcomes' (Qureshi and Harris, 2000, p 1). This definition thus seeks to differentiate between social care and health outcomes on the basis of being non-clinical and clinical respectively.

In health, outcome definitions have ranged from broad notions of 'a change in the *health status* of an individual, group or population which is attributable to a planned intervention or series of interventions, regardless of whether such an intervention was intended to change *health status*' (WHO, 1998, p 10, emphasis as in original document) to the more specific definitions within the United Kingdom (UK) Public Service Agreement 'to reduce substantially the mortality rates from major killers' and 'to narrow the health gap in childhood and throughout life between socio-economic groups and between the most deprived areas and the rest of the country' (DH, 2000, p 142). The Personal Social Services Research Unit (PSSRU) team (Forder et al, 2007) working for the Office for National Statistics (ONS, 2010) have drawn a useful parallel between the quality-adjusted life year (QALY) outcome measure used in health, 'which measures not only the extra life expectancy associated with a health care intervention but also the quality of those extra life years', with the Wanless (2006) review's 'activity of daily living adjusted year' (ADLAY) outcome, with its emphasis on 'the degree to which social care services improve people's functioning during the course of a year, such as being fed, clean, appropriately dressed, not socially excluded, feeling in control of one's life and so forth' (Forder et al, 2007, p 12). A comprehensive discussion of QALYs and the 'willingness to pay' monetary measures of quality in healthcare is outside the scope of this chapter and can be found in Baker et al (2008; see also Chapters Two and Three, this volume).

All of these definitions assume a linear model of planning and service delivery, which results in an individual experiencing an outcome (see Figure 7.1). They draw heavily on the production of welfare model (Donabedian, 1966; Audit Commission, 1986; Davies and Challis, 1986; Gaster, 1995; Nocon and Qureshi, 1996a, 1996b; Rouse, 1999; Challis et al, 2006), with its explicit relationship between inputs (resources), processes, outputs (services) and outcomes.

Figure 7.1: A linear approach to outcomes

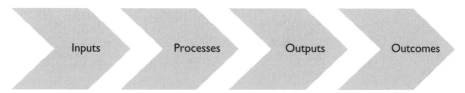

More recent frameworks of strategic commissioning have begun to question whether this model represents traditional public service incremental planning, with its inherent assumptions about top-down decision making about resources, processes and organisational service delivery. As such, the beneficiaries – individuals and communities – are viewed as being the recipients of services rather than being involved as co-producers not only in what gets provided but also, even more crucially, in which people-centred outcomes should be chosen at the start of the commissioning cycle. A reversed model creates a conceptual and practical shift to view the determination of outcomes as the starting point for considering appropriate services or other interventions that will improve specific aspects of people's well-being.

Such a shift aligns the process of strategic commissioning with that envisaged by the health and social care personalisation agenda, which aims 'to be the first public service reform programme which is co-produced, co-developed, co-evaluated and recognises that real change will only be achieved through the participation of users and carers at every stage' (HM Government, 2007, p 1; see also Chapter Eleven, this volume). It is also compatible with the vision for strategic commissioning set out by the Local Government Association and Confederation of British Industry:

> A strategic approach to commissioning and delivering community-based outcomes requires public bodies across a community to step back and take an overall view of their role in a locality. Leadership, here, is now more than just the management of services. It is about imagining

and delivering new solutions that do not yet exist, and being prepared for challenges yet to emerge. (LGA and CBI, 2008, p 5)

The suggestion here is that starting with outcomes encourages a 'zero-based' approach to strategic planning, one that makes no assumptions that current services are appropriate to realise the outcomes that matter to individuals and communities. It is the kind of thinking that led to the wholesale closure of institutional care for people with learning disabilities and mental health problems in the 1970s and 1980s and the move to community-based 'independence'. This approach will be explored further in a later section of this chapter but before that, it is important to examine how these relationships are expressed in models of the commissioning cycle.

Outcomes and the commissioning cycle

Outcome-based commissioning starts with the specification of user- or community-centred outcomes and then designs a procurement, monitoring and evaluation process that focuses on the achievement of these outcomes (see Figure 7.2).

Figure 7.2: Outcome-based commissioning cycle

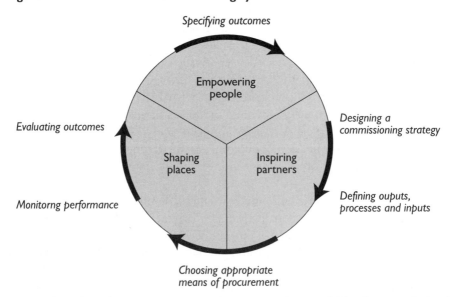

The philosophy of commissioning underpinning this model has been enshrined in a series of public policy guidance regarding health and social care with children and adults:

> Joint planning and commissioning is a tool for children's trusts – to
> build services around the needs of children and young people –

and to deliver their outcomes most efficiently and effectively. (HM Government, 2006, p 2)

The aim of this document is to help commissioners do this [focus on people] by showing how they can provide personalised services, promote health and well-being, proactively prevent ill health, and work in partnership to reduce health inequalities by focusing on outcomes for children and adults. (DH, 2007a, p 8)

World class commissioners will secure effective strategic capacity and capability to turn competence into excellence, transforming people's health and well-being outcomes at the local level, while reducing health inequalities and promoting inclusion. (DH, 2007b, p 3)

However, attempts to build outcomes into the commissioning process in this way, and particularly into the procurement process, are still relatively young and unproven. In particular, there are major theoretical and technical critiques of the limitations of the type of 'cause-and-effect' analysis that lies behind the outcomes–outputs–activities–inputs approach (Bovaird, 2008). Where the outcomes are themselves socially or publicly contestable (for example in relation to levels of risk experienced by children and young people or older people), the issues around outcome-based commissioning are even more contentious.

Outcome-based commissioning in health and social care is also being strongly promulgated through the personalisation agenda (HM Government, 2007) and the more recent framework for local authority commissioning for personalisation, which argues for the principle of 'ensuring that outcomes are at the centre of all developments designed to integrate commissioning and service delivery' (DH, 2008, p 16; DH, 2009). The coalition government elected in 2010 has announced its intention to promote this focus on outcomes by giving 'local communities greater control over public health budgets with payment by the outcomes they achieve in improving the health of local residents' (HM Government, 2010, p 28; see also Chapter Eleven, this volume).

One of the most advanced areas of outcome-based commissioning for public services was the Flexible New Deal programme (DWP, 2008), with its 'black box' approach to commissioning employment programmes. Providers were asked to deliver specific outcomes (usually jobs gained and held for a defined number of months) but, in principle, were able to decide themselves how best to achieve them. In this way, the Department for Work and Pensions (DWP) deliberately aimed to give providers the responsibility for determining the best ways to achieve outcomes to suit local circumstances. In practice, though, the House of Commons (2009) Select Committee noted that contract management arrangements were not quite in line with this aim, as DWP specified some activities that providers must make available to every customer, including an initial assessment of their barriers and needs; the agreement and regular review of a personalised work-focused action plan; and information about their rights and responsibilities on the programme.

The Department of Health approach to outcome-based commissioning has been much less 'black box' in its thinking. It expects primary care and hospital trusts to demonstrate some of the 'pathways' by means of which outcomes will be achieved and expects that the choice of these pathways in the commissioning process will be evidence based. As a consequence, there has been variable practice in health, with some primary care trusts (PCTs) attempting to make their commissioning highly outcome oriented, with as little prescription of 'pathways' as possible.

While outcome-based commissioning has been growing in importance in almost all public services in the UK, it is not clear whether this will result in outcome-based procurement. A review of service options might indicate which is likely to have the best outcomes, leading to a relatively traditional procurement process to secure that option. Still less is it clear that outcome-based commissioning will imply outcome-based contract payment mechanisms, since many factors that are likely to affect outcomes will be outside of the influence of the contractor. Nevertheless, experiments with more outcome-based procurement and contracting are indeed proceeding, to see how far they can sensibly be pushed and to explore the positive (and negative) behaviours to which they give rise.

Commissioners generally require to be convinced that providers bidding for contracts understand and have evidence for the pathways by means of which they hope to secure the outcomes that are being commissioned. Where there is good evidence of which pathways are most likely to work, commissioners need to consider whether to include this in the information given in the procurement process and in the tender evaluation process. Where commissioners are committed to a 'black box' approach, in which they give maximum discretion to providers, they may decide to forswear this approach, assuming that providers have picked up the information themselves in the marketplace (a rather risky assumption).

Providers involved in an outcome-based procurement process need to be able to show clearly how their processes give rise to, and assure, particular types of outcomes and particular levels of outcomes. Currently, this kind of analysis is only developed to a limited degree in most public services. Furthermore, providers need to indicate the risk levels attaching to the outcomes that are being commissioned. Insofar as the commissioning process leads to outcome-based contracts (and this approach has so far been quite rare), quite high-risk premiums may be demanded by providers where there is significant uncertainty about the factors influencing outcomes. Sometimes providers will be unprepared to take the full risk, whatever the risk premium.

The interrelationship between government prescriptions of strategic commissioning approaches with highly prescriptive performance management frameworks has thrown into question the extent to which the innovative outcome-focused approaches that strategic commissioning is meant to encourage are able to emerge in practice. For example, the political unacceptability of variation in the outcome performance of PCTs, the 'postcode lottery' phenomenon, led to the introduction of world class commissioning (NHS Information Centre, 2009) with its 11 competencies on which all PCTs were performance rated. It remains to be seen whether this results in reduced variation and greater prescription, and consequent uniformity – of outputs, processes and inputs of local patient pathways – especially with the more recent advent of clinical commissioning.

Outcome-focused commissioning: evidence from research

This section considers three research studies, two concerned with groups of adults and one with young people. The adult research was undertaken between 2003 and 2005 for two long-established voluntary organisations – Thomas Pocklington Trust, a national charity that works with people with a visual impairment, and MSA, a Midlands-based charity working with people with cerebral palsy (Willis et al, 2003, Willis and Wilson, 2004; Willis, 2005). In both cases, the researchers were asked to evaluate existing day services with a view to identifying a holistic understanding of users' needs and outcomes and how these might best be met. The researchers could have followed a service-focused methodology, identifying the outputs (services) that were being provided by the organisations and then evaluating the quality of life and quality of service experience dimensions. In contrast, the researchers chose to adopt an outcome-based approach, which started with a series of focus groups with users to explore their views on three broad outcome questions:

- 'safety': what enables you to feel safe within your own home and out and about in the community?
- 'happiness': what enables you to enjoy daily living within your own home and out and about in the community?
- 'development': what enables you to develop new ways of improving the quality of your life?

The aim of this approach was to elicit users' own definitions of the outcomes that were important to them as people living at home and in their neighbourhoods. For example, one person with visual impairment spoke about the pain and loss that he experienced when friends no longer greeted him after he became visually impaired and another expressed their annoyance that their relatives found it difficult to let them do things for themselves. People also talked about: the importance of telling friends about a bad day to "get it out of your system"; difficulties with going shopping and crossing the roads; and the lack of awareness among taxi drivers and public service staff of how to work with a visually impaired person.

People with cerebral palsy expressed similar views about: friendship and wanting more company; being able to access public transport; family and professionals taking the time "to understand what you feel and need"; and being treated as a person who can make decisions for themselves, "not a thing in a wheelchair". They also talked about the importance of living on their own with a personal assistant and "organisations and public buildings employing carers so that you can go to the swimming baths, theatre or restaurant".

From these responses, the researchers developed a set of statements, which summarised what each group of users felt enabled them to be safe and happy and to develop. These statements were then incorporated into a questionnaire, which was administered with a larger set of current users of both organisations, and for the visually impaired group, other people with a visual impairment who were not current users and staff from statutory and voluntary organisations who have an interest in working with visually impaired people. The aim was to discover which of the statements were most important to users and staff in order to determine user-focused strategic commissioning outcomes for each organisation (see Tables 7.1 and 7.2).

The importance of these findings is first that each group of people has distinct characteristics – it is not a case of one size fits all. This has significant implications for commissioning in that to specify the services and processes in contracts or other forms of procurement will inevitably limit outcome achievement. It supports the 'black box' New Deal approach to commissioning rather than a highly prescriptive specification of outputs, processes and inputs favoured in systems of inspection, star ratings and government by-performance targets (Bevan and Hood, 2006). Equally, it is an argument in favour of 'obligational' rather than 'arm's length' contractual relations (Sako, 1992).

Second, the rankings of the seven outcome enablers by the two groups of visually impaired people are broadly similar and contrast with some of the staff's responses. For example, both user groups ranked 'meeting people and friendship' as

Table 7.1: People with a visual impairment: rank order of responses

Outcome enabler	Existing users rating as very important (n=34)	Other people with visual impairment rating as very important (n=37)	Staff rating as important to all users (n=28)
Meeting people and friendship	1st	1st	5th
Getting information and advice about other services for people with a visual impairment	3rd	2nd	1st
Finding out about special equipment	5th	3rd	2nd
Having someone to talk to about your personal feelings	2nd	4th	7th
Building your confidence to go out and do things outside your home	6th	5th =	4th
Re-learning how to carry out everyday tasks in your home	7th	5th =	3rd
Getting help with practical everyday tasks	4th	7th	6th

Table 7.2: People with cerebral palsy: rank order of responses

Outcome enabler	Existing users rating as very important (*n*=18)
Access to leisure opportunities	1st
Information about services for people with a disability	2nd =
Opportunities to meet and support each other	2nd =
Someone to assist you in getting the things you need	4th
Building up your confidence to go out and do things outside your home	5th =
Access to educational opportunities	5th =
Opportunities to learn from each other's experience and knowledge	7th =
A personal assistant who would help you do what you want to do	7th =
Developing skills to do things for yourself	9th =
Adaptations to your homes to make them easier to live in	9th =
Access to employment opportunities	11th

their most important outcome enabler, whereas staff placed this fifth. Staff ranked 're-learning how to carry out everyday tasks in your home' as third whereas this is seventh and fifth in the two user group lists. How might such differences be explained?

One possibility is that long-term services for people with a visual impairment are not considered as a care management priority by many social care and related organisations. Thus, their focus is on the practicalities of information, equipment and doing things in the home, perhaps associated with rehabilitation relatively soon after sight loss, rather than longer-tem concerns such as social contact and talking about personal feelings. A second possibility is more fundamental. Oliver (1990) has argued that professionals tend to define outcomes in terms of people being able to care for themselves (cooking, washing, shopping and so on) whereas disabled people talk of being in control of their own lives and making choices. While these are not necessarily mutually exclusive, the differing emphasis may lead to contrasting 'world views' as demonstrated in the research findings.

Third, the responses of a number of the users in both studies reflected the social model of disability thesis that it is the way services are organised and run that disables people rather than their own individual characteristics. Thus, users suggested that taxi drivers, neighbours and shop staff, as well as professionals, needed to become aware of how they exclude users in day-to-day situations. One user thought that volunteers could act as "spontaneous sharers" by bringing what they see and read to life for those with visual impairment.

The overall implication of these studies is that the purposes and aims of commissioning should be expressed in terms of outcomes for people rather than services. Furthermore, the studies suggest that such outcomes should not only focus on individual needs but also promote wider agendas of counteracting social inclusion, reflecting the social model of disability. Examples from the research included awareness training for staff in leisure, libraries, supermarkets, restaurants and taxi firms as well as health and social care about how to understand the experience of, and positively involve, people with a sensory impairment or disability.

Commissioning for outcomes shifts the agenda away from a narrow focus on people's social care or health needs towards a broader understanding of what people require in order to become active citizens. As an example, a telling piece of mystery shopping was undertaken by 'older people researching the ability of councils to provide information on a range of mainstream services' (Audit Commission, 2008b, p 24). The topics of their enquiries bore a close resemblance to many of the key issues identified by users in the three research studies previously discussed: leisure and social activities; learning, employment and volunteering opportunities; and transport. The mystery shoppers found that 'they were commonly referred to adult social care, despite having no care needs' and the researchers concluded that councils should embrace a much broader role in ensuring 'that mainstream services are accessible to as many of the older people as possible, for as long as possible' (Audit Commission, 2008b, p 32). A number of local authorities have begun to develop such whole systems approaches to outcome-based commissioning. Wokingham Council's work to create a strategy written by, and for, older people to promote well-being and independence for residents as they grow older is a particularly fine example (Wokingham Borough Council, 2008).

This strategic focus on people-centred outcomes was also identified as an important variable in research to examine how local authorities and their partner organisations were commissioning positive activities for young people (PAYP) (Willis et al, 2008). PAYP was introduced in 2003 as a targeted three-year cross-departmental programme for young people aged 8-19 at risk of committing a crime or becoming socially excluded. In 2007, the government broadened the scope of the strategy by arguing that 'participation in constructive leisure-time activities, particularly those that are sustained through the teenage years, can have a significant impact on young people's resilience and outcomes in later life' (HM Treasury, 2007, p 6). This shift reflects the development of thinking from services designed to tackle problem-defined needs to wider whole-population outcome commissioning.

The research aimed to explore how local authorities and their partners had responded to this strategy and took place in 17 local authorities across three government regions. In addition to documentary and questionnaire analysis, focus group discussions were held with young people and key stakeholders in six case study local authorities. The wide variation in approaches adopted by different local authorities was striking. While some were working with a handful of partners focusing on a limited number of young people who were involved in antisocial and other disruptive behaviour, others had mapped nearly three hundred organisations providing youth activities. For the former, partnerships were confined to local authority, police, education and health agencies; in the latter there was a wider representation of voluntary, community and private sector organisations. Some had developed highly participative processes of involving young people in all the stages of the commissioning cycle (planning outcomes, procuring, monitoring and evaluating) while others focused on more limited consultative mechanisms.

Perhaps the most revealing variation was how authorities approached procurement. Some defined procurement as essentially concerned with the 'make or buy' choice with its emphasis on the provision of services either in-house or by contracting with external providers to meet identified need. Such thinking is in line with many of the theoretical and policy-based models of commissioning previously discussed in this chapter. At their extreme, the terms 'commissioning', 'procurement' and 'contracting' become interchangeable. Other authorities drew a distinction between 'commissioning' as a strategic activity (DH, 2009; CSP, 2010), 'procurement' as the process of choosing the appropriate means to achieve defined people-centred outcomes and 'contracting' as one of a range of ways of producing outputs that are designed to deliver those outcomes. The resulting model of strategic commissioning for outcomes can be expressed as shown in Figure 7.3.

This model recognises that there is a wide range of options open to local authorities, NHS organisations and others in considering how to achieve outcomes through the process of strategic commissioning and procurement. Some of these options involve the allocation of financial resources while others depend more on influence and networks. Given the severe financial restraints that will be placed on public spending budgets over the next five years, commissioning bodies will need to create imaginative solutions working with public, voluntary and private organisations and communities and individuals that do not require large budgets. Such approaches will be explored further in the final section of this chapter.

Figure 7.3: Outcome-based commissioning

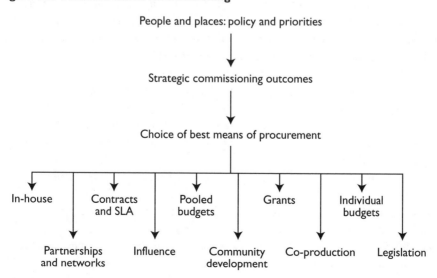

Conclusion: outcomes and strategic commissioning futures in a receding state

Whatever the level of cuts in public spending over the next few years, the overriding picture will be of increased demand for social care and health services chasing reduced public supply. The stark consequence will be that many more people will be left to fend for themselves, particularly in relation to the social care of people with physical and learning disabilities, mental health problems and older people. However, this does not mean that there is no role for commissioning but suggests that it will change from an emphasis on procuring services through contracts, grants and individual budgets to the more 'devolved' options identified on the bottom line of this outcome-based commissioning model. One formulation of this has been expounded by the Prime Minister David Cameron in his 'Big Society' concept:

> You can call it liberalism. You can call it empowerment. You can call it freedom. You can call it responsibility. I call it the Big Society. The Big Society is about a huge culture change where people, in their everyday lives, in their homes, in their neighbourhoods, in their workplace don't always turn to officials, local authorities or central government for answers to the problems they face but instead feel both free and powerful enough to help themselves and their own communities. (Cameron, 2010)

Another, rather different expression of this idea is found in work on 'co-production'. This concept has been a slow burner in the public sector, from its early appearance in public administration in the United States in the 1980s, through increasing usage in development economics in the 1980s and 1990s, to its increasing usage in countries of the Organisation for Economic Co-operation and Development in the last decade (Bovaird, 2007). The concept is very elastic and has been used to cover all of the following elements of engagement by users and communities in public management decisions:

- co-planning of policy – for example, deliberative participation, Planning for Real, Open Space;
- co-design of services – for example, user consultation, innovation labs;
- co-commissioning services – for example, devolved grant systems, community chest, individual budgets;
- co-financing services – for example, fundraising, charges, agreement to tax increases;
- co-managing services – for example, leisure centre trusts, community management of public assets;
- co-delivery of services – for example, expert patients, volunteer firefighters, Neighbourhood Watch;

- co-monitoring and co-evaluation of services – for example, user ratings, citizen inspectors.

As this suggests, the co-production approach includes co-commissioning, where public agencies actually engage users and communities within the commissioning approach itself. The most obvious example of this is direct payments in social services, or more generally individual budgets, where users have the opportunity to decide for themselves what services they receive with public sector budgets (see Chapter Eleven, this volume). However, the co-commissioning approach has also spread to other arenas; for example, in its initiative 'Aiming High for Young People', the New Labour government proposed increasing young people's direct control and influence, so that by 2018 they would be actively shaping decisions on at least 25% of local authorities' budgets for positive activities.

However, more commonly, commissioners can build co-production into the services that they commission. Perhaps the best-known example of this in the UK is in social services in the London Borough of Camden, where commissioners and service providers worked with the new economics foundation on its 'Sustainable Commissioning Model' to draw up a service specification based on co-production. The tender (nef, nd) specified that: 'We would encourage providers to adopt the model of "co-production" whereby services are planned and delivered in mutually beneficial ways that acknowledge and reward local "lay" experience while continuing to value professional expertise. Service users should be regarded as an asset and encouraged to work alongside professionals as partners in the delivery of services' and that 'the service should be delivered in partnership with service users'. The successful consortium of providers has been providing the re-commissioned day care service since the beginning of October 2007.

A different approach to devolving delivery of commissioned services is evidenced in experiments in partnership working, which have encouraged unexpected community development initiatives. The Gloucestershire Village Agents project started life with the aim of providing a coordinated electronic information service for older people living in isolated rural communities. Over time, it morphed into a sophisticated support network that was able to help people to cope during severe flooding; to negotiate changes to bus routes; to set up an internet café and assist with online shopping; and to arrange activities in village halls and pubs (Callinan, 2008; Wilson et al, 2008). Its success has motivated similar projects in Cumbria, Essex, Northamptonshire and Somerset. Village Agents was one of eight DWP LinkAge Plus pilot projects working with older people, which inspired a creative variety of capacity-building initiatives involving commissioning partnerships between councils, health, private, community and voluntary organisations (Willis and Dalziel, 2009).

Finally, the Total Place policy in the last year of New Labour's term in office encouraged pilot areas to consider how whole community commissioning, bringing together the resources and ideas of all statutory organisations working in a defined local area, might enable the achievement of better outcomes and community empowerment as well as resource efficiencies. The concluding report reflects the outcome-based commissioning approach outlined in this chapter: 'Making the shift from the commissioning and procurement of a defined product or service, to engaging the supply side in developing solutions to outcomes, can fully release the expertise and innovation of suppliers to develop new and more effective approaches – and delivers more for less' (HM Treasury and DCLG, 2010, p 43).

Initial pronouncements from the incoming coalition government provide support for the argument that outcome-based commissioning will continue to be a key tool of public policy. As the local government minister has said, 'whatever we call the next generation of Total Place, it has to be about outcomes. The challenge now isn't about talking but about delivery on the ground' (Neill, 2010). This chapter has sought to identify the opportunities for statutory sector commissioners and their partners in private, voluntary and community organisations to create positive ways of responding to this challenge. In the context of a receding state, the consequence of not seizing these opportunities will be poorer outcomes for individuals and communities.

Further reading

Key sources include:

- Bovaird, T. (2007) 'Beyond engagement and participation – user and community co-production of public services', *Public Administration Review*, vol 67, no 5, pp 846–60.
- Davies, H., Nutley, S. and Smith, P. (eds) (2000) *What works? Evidence-based policy and practice in public services*, Bristol: The Policy Press.
- Gaster, L. and Squires, A. (eds) (2003) *Providing quality in the public sector*, Buckingham: Open University Press.
- Shaping Our Lives (2003) *Social services users' own definitions of quality outcomes*, York: Joseph Rowntree Foundation.

Useful websites

- Centre for Excellence and Outcomes in Children's and Young People's Services: www.c4eo.org.uk/
- Clinical and Health Outcomes Knowledge Base: www.nchod.nhs.uk/
- Commissioning Support Organisation: www.commissioningsupport.org.uk/
- Dartington Social Research Unit: www.dartington.org.uk/
- DH Care Networks: www.dhcarenetworks.org.uk/
- Governance International: www.govint.org/
- Fiscal Policy Studies Institute: www.resultsaccountability.com/
- Health Investment Network: www.networks.nhs.uk/nhs-networks/health-investment-network

- Joseph Rowntree Foundation: www.jrf.org.uk/
- National Commissioning and Contracting Conference: www.publicsectorconferences.co.uk/index.htm
- Social Policy Research Unit, University of York: www.york.ac.uk/inst/spru/

Reflective exercises

1. Make a list of the most important ways in which your performance at work is measured and managed. Include both organisational and personal indicators, targets and standards. How much do these performance measures tell you about whether individuals, communities or citizens benefit from what you and your colleagues and partners do? What do service users say matters to them in terms of the quality of their lives?
2. Think about what is important to you about your own health and that of your close family and friends. Define relevant 'safety', 'happiness' and 'development' health outcomes. Choose one of these outcomes and consider what key outputs (services), processes and inputs (resources) are needed to ensure its achievement. Sketch an outcome-based commissioning pathway for your chosen outcome:

> **Outcome ⟶ Outputs ⟶ Processes ⟶ Inputs**
> *(There may be several outputs, processes and inputs required to achieve your chosen outcome)*

3. Who is responsible in your organisation or partnership for each of the nine dimensions of the outcome-based commissioning cycle model (see above)? How can the coordination of these functions be improved to assure the achievement of people-centred commissioning outcomes?
4. Consider an aspect of your organisation's current procurement practice designed to achieve a people-centred outcome. How might the range of procurement options be widened? What other organisations and community groups would need to be involved as a result?

References

Audit Commission (1986) *Performance review in local government*, London: HMSO.

Audit Commission (2008a) *Are we there yet? Improving governance and resource management in children's trusts*, London: Audit Commission.

Audit Commission (2008b) *Don't stop me now: preparing for an ageing population*, London: Audit Commission.

Audit Commission and SSI (Social Services Inspectorate) (1999) *Making connections: learning the lessons from Joint Reviews 1998/9*, London: Audit Commission.

Audit Commission and SSI (2000) *Promising prospects: learning the lessons from Joint Reviews 1999/2000 English authorities*, London: Audit Commission.

Baker, R., Mason, H., Donaldson, C. and Jones-Lee, M. (2008) 'Valuing public sector outputs', in J. Hartley, C. Donaldson, C. Squelcher and M. Wallace (eds) *Managing to improve public services*, Cambridge: Cambridge University Press, pp 153-75.

Bevan, G. and Hood, C. (2006) 'What's measured is what matters: targets and gaming in the English public health care system', *Public Administration*, vol 84, no 3, pp 517-38.

Bovaird, T. (2007) 'Beyond engagement and participation – user and community co-production of public services', *Public Administration Review*, vol 67, no 5, pp 846-60.

Bovaird, T. (2008) 'Emergent strategic management and planning mechanisms in complex adaptive systems: the case of the UK Best Value initiative', *Public Management Review*, vol 10, no 3, pp 319-40.

Bovaird, T. and Löffler, E. (2003) 'Evaluating the quality of public governance: indicators, models and methodologies', *International Review of Administrative Sciences*, vol 69, no 3, pp 313-28.

Bovaird, T. and Löffler, E. (eds) (2009) *Public management and governance* (2nd edition), London: Routledge.

Callinan, R. (2008) *LinkAge Plus: end of project report: Village Agents*, Gloucestershire County Council and Gloucestershire Rural Community Council, www.villageagents.org.uk/downloads/LinkAge%20Plus.doc

Cameron, D. (2010) Big Society speech, 19 July, www.number10.gov.uk/news/speeches-and-transcripts/2010/07/big-society-speech-53572

Challis, D., Clarkson, P. and Warburton, R. (2006) *Performance indicators in social care for older people*, Aldershot: Ashgate.

Clarke, J. and Glendinning, C. (2002) 'Partnership and the remaking of welfare governance', in C. Glendinning, M. Powell and K. Rummery (eds) *Partnerships, New Labour and the governance of welfare*, Bristol: The Policy Press, pp 33-50.

CSP (2010) *Commissioning support programme*, http://www.commissioningsupport.org.uk/

Darzi, A. (2008) 'Summary letter: our NHS – secured today for future generations', in Department of Health *High quality care for all: NHS next stage review final report*, London: Department of Health.

Davies, B. and Challis, D. (1986) *Matching resources to needs in community care*, Aldershot: Gower.

Davies, H., Nutley, S. and Smith, P. (eds) (2000) *What works? Evidence-based policy and practice in public services*, Bristol: The Policy Press.

DH (Department of Health) (2000) *The NHS plan: a plan for investment, a plan for reform*, London: TSO.

DH (2003) *The Victoria Climbié inquiry: summary report*, London: DH.

DH (2004) *Practice-based commissioning: engaging practices in commissioning*, London: DH.

DH (2005) *Independence, well-being and choice: our vision for the future for social care for adults in England*, London: DH.

DH (2007a) *Commissioning framework for health and well-being*, London: DH.

DH (2007b) *NHS world class commissioning competencies*, Gateway Reference 8754, London: DH, http://www.dh.gov.uk/prod_consum_dh/groups/dh_digitalassets/@dh/@en/documents/digitalasset/dh_080964.pdf

DH (2008) *Commissioning for personalisation: a framework for local authority commissioners*, London: DH.

DH (2009) *Commissioning and contracting for outcomes: care services efficiency delivery*, London: DH, www.dhcarenetworks.org.uk/_library/Resources/CSED/CSEDProduct/Contracting_for_Outcomes_v04_00_MCF_20Apr09.pdf

Donabedian, A. (1966) 'Evaluating the quality of medical care', *Millbank Memorial Fund Quarterly*, vol 4, pp 166-206.

Donabedian, A. (1980, 1982, 1985) *Explorations in quality assessment and monitoring, vol 1: the definition of quality and approaches to its assessment, vol 2: the criteria and standards of quality, vol 3: the methods and findings of quality assessment and monitoring*, Ann Arbor, MI: Health Administration Press.

DWP (Department for Work and Pensions) (2008) *Transforming Britain's labour market: ten years of the new deal*, London: DWP.

Forder, J., Netten, A., Caiels, J., Smith, J. and Malley, J. (2007) *Measuring outcomes in social care: conceptual development and empirical design: quality measurement framework project*, Discussion Paper 2422, Canterbury: PSSRU, University of Kent.

Gaster, L. (1995) *Quality in public services*, Buckingham: Open University Press.

Gaster, L. and Squires, A. (eds) (2003) *Providing quality in the public sector*, Buckingham: Open University Press.

HM Government (2005) *Opportunity age: meeting the challenges of ageing in the 21st century*, London: HM Government.

HM Government (2006) *Joint planning and commissioning framework for children, young people and maternity services*, London: Department for Education and Skills and Department of Health.

HM Government (2007) *Putting People First: a shared commitment to the transformation of adult social care*, London: DH.

HM Government (2010) *The coalition: our programme for government*, London: Cabinet Office.

HM Treasury (2003) *Every child matters*, London: TSO.

HM Treasury (2007) *Aiming high for young people: a ten-year strategy for positive activities*, London: HM Treasury and DCSF.

HM Treasury and DCLG (Department for Communities and Local Government) (2010) *Total place: a whole area approach to public services*, London: HM Treasury.

House of Commons (2009) *DWP's commissioning strategy and the flexible New Deal*, London: Work and Pensions Committee, www.parliament.uk/search/results/?q=Flexible+New+Deal

Knapp, M., Wistow, G. and Jones, N. (1992) 'Smart moves', *Health Services Journal*, 29 October, pp. 28-30.

LGA and CBI (Local Government Association and Confederation of British Industry) (2008) *Improving the strategic commissioning of public services: a joint LGA/CBI vision*, London: LGA, http://publicservices.cbi.org.uk/uploaded/Improving_strategic_commissioning.pdf

Means, R., Richards, S. and Smith, R. (2003) *Community care: policy and practice* (3rd edition), Basingstoke: Palgrave Macmillan.

Morgan, C. and Murgatroyd, S. (1994) *Total quality management in the public sector: an international perspective*, Buckingham: Open University Press.

NCC (National Consumer Council) (1986) *Measuring up: consumer assessment of local authority services: guideline study*, London: NCC.

nef (new economics foundation) (nd) *Commissioning for co-production in Camden*, London: nef, www.socialinclusion.org.uk/publications/CommissioningCoproduction.pdf

Neill, B. (2010) Speech at a Leadership Centre for Local Government dinner, 20 May, quoted in M. Burton 'Government to retain "principle of Total Place"', 26 May, www.localgov.co.uk/index.cfm?method=news.detail&id=89149

NHS Information Centre (2009) *Information for world class commissioning*, London: NHS Information Centre, www.ic.nhs.uk/commissioning

Nocon, A. and Qureshi, H. (1996a) *Outcomes of community care for users and carers: a social services perspective*, Buckingham: Open University Press.

Nocon, A. and Qureshi, H. (1996b) 'Outcome measurement in community care', in P. Smith (ed) *Measuring outcome in the public sector*, London: Taylor & Francis, pp 74-83.

Oliver, M. (1990) *The politics of disablement*, Basingstoke: Macmillan.

ONS (Office for National Statistics) (2010) *Measuring outcomes for public service users: final report*, London: ONS, www.ons.gov.uk/about-statistics/methodology-and-quality/measuring-outcomes-for-public-service-users/mopsu-reports-and-updates/index.html

Parker, R., Ward, H., Jackson, S., Aldgate, J. and Wedge, P. (eds) (1991) *Looking after children: assessing outcomes in child care*, London: HMSO.

Peters, T. and Waterman, R. (1982) *In search of excellence: lessons from America's best run companies*, New York, NY: Harper & Row.

Qureshi, H. (2000) 'Outcomes and assessment with older people', *Research Works*, York: Social Policy Research Unit.

Qureshi, H. and Harris, J. (2000) 'Identifying stakeholder views about the outcomes of social care, and using outcome concepts in practice and user surveys', Paper presented at *Intsoceval* workshop 2000, Verwey-Jonker Institute, Utrecht, www.intsocevalorg/files/utrecht/Qureshi.pdf

Richardson, F. (2006) 'Introduction: the commissioning context', in Care Services Improvement Partnership *Commissioning eBook,* www.dhcarenetworks.org.uk/_library/Chap1FRichardson.pdf

Rouse, J. (1999) 'Performance management, quality management and contracts', in S. Horton and D. Farnham (eds) *Public management in Britain*, Basingstoke: Macmillan, pp 76-93.

Sako, M. (1992) *Prices, quality and trust: inter-firm relations in Britain and Japan*, Cambridge: Cambridge University Press.

Shaping Our Lives (2003) *Social services users' own definitions of quality outcomes*, York: Joseph Rowntree Foundation.

Skelcher, C. (1992) *Managing for service quality*, Harlow: Longman.

Smith, P. (1996) 'A framework for analysing the measurement of outcome', in P. Smith (ed) *Measuring outcome in the public sector*, London: Taylor & Francis, pp 1-19.

Wanless, D. (2006) *Securing good care for older people: taking a long term view*, London: King's Fund.

WHO (World Health Organization) (1998) *Health promotion glossary*, Geneva: WHO.

Willis, M. (2005) 'Defining vision', *Community Care*, 7 July, pp 32-3.

Willis, M. and Dalziel, R. (2009) *LinkAge Plus: capacity building – enabling and empowering older people as independent and active citizens*, Research Report No 571, London: Department for Work and Pensions, http://campaigns.dwp.gov.uk/asd/asd5/rports2009-2010/rrep571.pdf

Willis, M. and Wilson, L. (2004) *Evaluation of MSA for Midland people with cerebral palsy: final research report*, Birmingham: INLOGOV, University of Birmingham.

Willis, M. H., Douglas, G. G. A., Dunstan, E. and Pavey, S. (2003) *Evaluation of Pocklington day services in the West Midlands: final research report for Thomas Pocklington Trust*, Birmingham: INLOGOV and VICTAR, University of Birmingham.

Willis, M., Jimpson, G., Dalziel, R. and Ali, J. (2008) *Commissioning positive activities for young people*, Leicester: National Youth Agency.

Wilson, L., Crow, A. and Willis, M. (2008) *Linkage Plus project: Village Agents – an evaluation*, Birmingham: INLOGOV, University of Birmingham.

Wokingham Borough Council (2008) *Young at heart: a strategy to promote wellbeing and independence for residents of Wokingham Borough as they grow older 2008 to 2018*, Wokingham: Wokingham Borough Council, www.wokingham.gov.uk/health-social-care/older/strategy-older-people/

Part Two

Key themes

EIGHT

The economics of commissioning

Peter Watt

Summary

This chapter explores:
- key concepts from economics that influence the commissioning process;
- the role of commissioning in relation to the service user;
- the role of commissioning in relation to suppliers;
- a combination of theoretical and practical insights into the economics of commissioning.

This chapter discusses a range of economic considerations that are relevant to commissioning. There is a clear economic role for the commissioning function, but the extent to which it should reside in public sector organisations and the extent to which it should be more widely dispersed are currently evolving (see also the Introduction to this book and Chapter One; this chapter also links to arguments developed by Chris Lonsdale in Chapter Four). Commissioners have a role both in relation to the consumer of public services and also in relation to the supplier of services. In relation to the *consumer*, commissioners may work with the market to help consumers get what they want. Commissioners may have a role if the consumer is making the 'wrong choices', although this is controversial, and there are also many ways in which the market can fail where commissioning can play a role. In relation to the *supplier*, commissioners make strategic make-or-buy decisions and also have a role in contractual relations.

This chapter begins with a discussion of the commissioner in relation to the consumer or service user and looks first at the question of consumer sovereignty – one of the basic value judgements underlying economics. Consumer sovereignty reflects the view that each person is the best judge of what is good for their well-being. An implication is that it is therefore good to organise society in a way that gives people what they want, 'within the constraints imposed by other people being free to get what they want' (Sugden, 2004, p 1016). Another part of this view, as expressed by Adam Smith (1930 [1776], p 625, cited in Persky, 1993), is that services should be consumer-led, rather than provider-led: 'Consumption is the sole end and purpose of all production; and the interests of the producer ought to be attended to, only so far as it may be necessary for promoting that of the consumer.' These assumptions about consumption lead to a powerful endorsement of the market as a way of organising society, formalised in what is called the first fundamental theorem of welfare economics: that competitive markets lead to an optimum allocation of resources (Arrow and Debreu, 1954). Although such optimal qualities provide the reason why economists generally have a preference for market forms of organisation, there will always be a need for government to provide conditions for the market to work by enforcing property rights and preventing theft. In addition to this fundamental 'law-and-order and property rights' role for government, there is also a case for considering government intervention in cases where the market may fail to operate optimally. Identifying such cases provides the basis for the 'market failure' arguments for government activity. Thus, we can consider the consumer side of commissioning by posing two questions: first, what is the role of commissioning under a pure market system, and second, what is the role of commissioning when the market fails?

Commissioning roles in a market system

Helping the user to satisfy their preferences

If society is organised by a pure laissez-faire system of market freedom, is there any role for commissioning? Should not people just decide what goods and services they want and buy them without the need for any intermediaries? In examining this question it is interesting to consider a hierarchy of types of spending as discussed by Friedman and Friedman (1980) and set out in Table 8.1. In the table the top left-hand box shows a person spending their own money on themselves. In this case they would have every incentive to get value for money (VFM). In the top right-hand box they are spending their own money on someone else, and in this case have an incentive to economise, but not necessarily to get something good – at least as judged by the recipient.[1] In the bottom left-hand box they are spending someone else's money on themselves and they have an incentive to get something good but not necessarily keep the expense down. Last, in the bottom right-hand box they are spending someone else's money on someone else, and they have an incentive neither to get something good nor to keep the expense

Table 8.1: Different types of spending

Whose money?	On whom spent?	
	You	Someone else
Yours	Shopping – incentive to get VFM	For example, a present. Incentive to economise but not to get VFM – at least as judged by the recipient
Someone else's	Expense account – incentive to get good VFM, but not to keep spending down	Little incentive to economise or to get good VFM for the recipient

Source: Adapted from Friedman and Friedman (1980, pp 116-17)

down. Commissioning falls into the bottom right-hand box and at first sight would seem to have no place in a sensible system. For example, discussing social care, Glasby et al (2009, p 482) argue that 'it seems as though direct payment recipients have more of vested interest than the local authority in ensuring that each pound available is spent as effectively as possible and in designing support that enables them to have greater choice and control over their own lives'.

Why, then, have an intermediary or middleman buy services for you when you can do it yourself? The reason for using an intermediary fits in with the usual reason for trading in a market – employ an intermediary when they can carry out the task more cost-effectively than you can yourself. Thus, customers may choose to buy via an agent, rather than direct from the producer. Also, producers of services may often choose to sell via retailers, rather than direct to the customer. Intermediaries will be used when found to be cost-effective, as tested by the market. We now discuss the role of intermediaries in more detail.

The commissioner as customer representative

Stinchcombe (1984, p 863) identifies three types of customer agents – retailers, personal representatives and professionals. Retailers bring together the products of primary producers in a convenient location and supply some expertise. In a competitive market they rely on producers and consumers choosing to use them. They charge for their services but competition constrains them to provide value for money. In the same way, a consumer may ask a personal representative to act on their behalf when they wish to buy services instead of going direct to the supplier. Examples include insurance brokers, financial advisers and hotel booking agencies. Recipients of direct payments may wish to have someone represent or help with representing their interests.

Why might a buyer want to buy via a personal representative? They may want to do so because what they are buying is complex and they may wish for help in understanding what they want and in controlling the supplier. An important insight into this question is supplied by principal-agent theory (Ross, 1973; Jensen and Meckling, 1976; Sappington, 1991). Principal-agent theory examines the issues that arise when a principal buys the services of an agent. The principal might be a consumer and the agent a supplier, or the principal might be an employer and the agent an employee. Principal-agent theory notes that the objectives of the principal and the agent will generally differ. In medicine, one manifestation of the problem has been labelled 'supplier-induced demand' (Evans, 1974, 1976). The buyer of a service will want to get the maximum quality and quantity they can for their money and will have preferences about the way the service is provided, whereas the supplier may opportunistically seek to provide the minimum (Williamson, 1975, p 26) and may want to provide the service in the way that suits them rather than the buyer. For example, in social care, scheduling of visits may be 'with limited regard for recipient preferences about when help is most needed' (Benjamin and Fennell, 2007, p 354). Here, self-directed support, backed by the direct power of the purse, is likely to aid rather than hinder the social care user in getting the care they want. Research so far suggests that this is the case (Glasby and Littlechild, 2009; see also Chapter Eleven, this volume).

As well as the problem of the agent's different objectives, a further problem for the principal is that the agent is likely to have better knowledge of what they are supplying than the principal. This differential knowledge may not always be a great problem in social care where aspects of a service such as home care may not be particularly recondite. Nevertheless, very many recipients of social care are 'vulnerable' in some sense so the problem should not be dismissed. Problems of differential knowledge can be more severe in other areas, such as healthcare – although recently the internet has offered some mitigation of the problem of dealing with experts. In economics, differential knowledge comes under the general heading of *information asymmetry* (Milgrom and Roberts, 1992, pp 140-3). Information asymmetry generates difficult problems, not least because an important reason for getting someone to carry out a task is that they are an expert. But because they *are* an expert it is more difficult for the principal to control the transaction (Dulleck and Kerschbamer, 2006). For example, in healthcare the principal (patient) often cannot tell whether they need the services of a doctor. In principal-agent theory, this is called the problem of *hidden information*. In addition, the patient cannot observe how much effort a doctor puts into their care. This is called the problem of *hidden action* (Milgrom and Roberts, 1992, pp 140-3; De Jaegher, 2010, p 124). These problems of hidden information and hidden action are not restricted to healthcare but also apply to the more complex aspects of social care. Financial services generate similar issues, which occur generally in markets where information is important.

We can see from this discussion that in healthcare the principal may have problems in controlling the agent, in the sense of knowing whether they need healthcare and knowing how good the care is that they have received. This may also, to an extent, be a problem in other areas such as education. One possible solution is for the principal to get help with the problem from a personal representative or commissioner of the service.[2] But if they have difficulty controlling the healthcare-providing agent, will not the same difficulties apply to controlling their personal representative?

Some important insights into this problem were provided by Darby and Karni (1973) in their analysis of what they labelled *credence goods*:

> Credence qualities are those which, although worthwhile, cannot be evaluated in normal use. Instead the assessment of their value requires additional costly information. An example would be the claimed advantages of the removal of an appendix, which will be correct or not according to whether the organ is diseased. The purchaser will have no different experience after the operation whether or not the organ was diseased. (Darby and Karni, 1973, p 69)

A useful technique for reducing the scope that credence goods afford for opportunism by experts is to split up the task so that one provider has the task of deciding what is required and a different provider has the task of actually supplying it. A similar approach is to pay one expert to provide a service and pay a second expert, the commissioner, to monitor the necessity for the service and its quality. Such a split may control the incentive to recommend unnecessary services that can be present when one supplier carries out both tasks and may hence have a conflict of interests. The agent carrying out diagnosis does not have the same incentive as the provider of the service to recommend unnecessary treatment. In local government, there has long been an awareness that the client–contractor split is likely to reduce the extent to which services are provider led (Stewart and Walsh, 1992), although there is also an awareness that such separation can be costly (House of Commons Health Committee, 2010, p 15).

Although separating diagnosis and treatment has the benefit of reducing the extent to which services are likely to be provider led, that does not mean that it is always worthwhile to separate diagnosis and treatment as there are likely to be considerable *economies of scope* between diagnosis and treatment. Economies of scope occur when the total cost of two tasks carried out together are less than when they are carried out separately. An example would be the benefit of bringing together the task of dismantling a car's clutch for diagnostic purposes and the task of replacing the clutch plate. Similarly, it may be costly for all concerned to carry out a separate diagnostic operation on a patient that finds a diseased appendix from a subsequent operation to remove it (Darby and Karni, 1973). In social care there is a cost to separating assessment of need from the subsequent actions designed to address that need. When we visit a shop or a restaurant we usually consider advice from the shopkeeper or waiter even though we understand that the advice may not be disinterested. The benefits of economies of scope are likely to outweigh provider-led aspects of the advice we receive, but it can be a fine balance. For the same reason, a professional 'independent support broker' role for social care seems unlikely to be cost-effective (Duffy and Fulton, 2009). If service users have control of a personal budget, they can decide for themselves whether they want to purchase any brokerage, although it may be only from costly experience that they will know whether or not they needed to purchase brokerage.

At times, information problems for the service user can be very considerable. Although the above discussion has been in terms of a patient not knowing whether or not they are in need of a *cure* from a doctor, and not being able to tell fully how much effort has gone into supplying that cure, the market for prevention may be even more problematic, as knowing whether or not one is in need of a cure is generally an easier problem than knowing whether or not one is in need of prevention.

When a patient seeks a cure they at least have information that they feel unwell and can also observe whether that feeling has gone after they have received the services of a doctor. With prevention, however, the information asymmetries are compounded. The patient is, instead, trying to ascertain whether, in the absence of preventive services, they will feel unwell in the future, and subsequently whether their health state has or has not benefited from these preventive services. They may well then welcome the expertise of a commissioner in navigating such difficulties. Such problems can be magnified when preventive care is funded by social care budgets and curative services are funded by healthcare budgets. This kind of organisational structure can lead to misallocation of resources to the detriment of prevention, in cases where nevertheless prevention is more cost-effective than cure (see Chapter Ten, this volume, for further discussion of joint commissioning).

One way of bringing diagnosis and treatment together to obtain economies of scope is to entrust a member of a profession with both tasks. The professional is given the role of providing both the service and self-monitoring. However, there have long been doubts about the wisdom of relying entirely on this mechanism. George Bernard Shaw wrote in 1906 that 'all professions are conspiracies against the laity' (Shaw, 1930 [1906], Act 1) and more recently it was found to be a resounding mistake to place such trust in Dr Harold Shipman.

From this discussion we can see that a demand for commissioning services may arise in a purely private market to assist the customer by providing elements of expertise, diagnosis and the monitoring of quality, when services are in the form of credence goods.

Commissioning of services may also arise in conjunction with *insurance*. Because the need for health and personal care may be unpredictable and random, and can impose heavy loss, it may be attractive to purchase insurance as, analogously, it may be attractive to purchase insurance against motoring accidents. The insurance company may then take on the role of commissioning the care and controlling the expert provider – be it the car repair shop or the surgeon, although 'even expert collective purchasers of health services, such as insurance organisations, find it difficult to judge whether services are being provided according to their preferences' (Smith et al, 1997, p 39). And this problem of controlling the expert provider is likely to extend to general practitioner consortia employing 'expert commissioners' on their behalf, as consortia will have the problem of judging whether the commissioners have purchased efficiently.

Failure of preferences?

So far we have looked at the role of the commissioner in the scenario where markets are working to deliver what people want. This approach is based on the value judgement that delivering what people want is an appropriate objective. This does not imply that each person is a perfect judge of what makes them happy but, rather, that it may be difficult to find an agent to do this that is likely consistently to do it better. Winston Churchill (1947) expressed a similar view about democracy: 'No one pretends that democracy is perfect or all-wise. Indeed, it has been said that democracy is the worst form of government except all those other forms that have been tried from time to time.' The question is – is it sensible to argue that people cannot make their own choices? Lerner (1972, p 258) notes that 'one of the deepest scars of my early youth was etched when my teacher told me, "You do not want that," after I had told her that I did'. The idea that the market may be delivering according to people's preferences, but that those preferences could be wrong, underlies Musgrave's (1959) conception of 'merit wants': goods and services that people should want even if they don't. Musgrave (1959, p 14) argued that:

> A case for the satisfaction of merit wants and for interference with consumer sovereignty, narrowly defined, may derive from the role of leadership in a democratic society. While consumer sovereignty is the general rule, situations may arise, within the context of a democratic community, where an informed group is justified in imposing its decision on others. Few will deny there is a case for regulating the sale of drugs or for providing certain health facilities. The advantages of education are more evident to the informed than the uninformed, thus justifying compulsion in the allocation of resources to education; interference in the preference patterns of families may be directed at protecting the interest of minors; the freedom to belong may override the freedom to exclude, and so forth.

However, the concept of 'merit wants' is problematic, because those same people who are assumed to have 'incorrect preferences' are also voting to choose the government that is assumed to know better. Musgrave himself recognises the problem: 'The concept of merit or demerit goods, to be sure, must be viewed with caution because it may serve as a vehicle for totalitarian rule' (Musgrave and Musgrave, 1989, p 58).

Over the last century, views have moved from a fairly ready willingness to overturn consumer sovereignty to a concern to avoid that wherever possible. Douglas Jay expressed clear paternalist sentiments in 1937: 'In the case of nutrition and health, just as in the case of education, the gentleman in Whitehall really does know better what is good for people than the people know themselves' (Jay, 1937, p 317, cited in Toye, 2002, p 187). Eighty years later, these views contrast strongly with the government's view on the desirability of person–centred adult social care in 2007:

> The time has now come to build on best practice and replace paternalistic, reactive care of variable quality with a mainstream system focussed on prevention, early intervention, enablement, and high quality personally tailored services. In the future, we want people to have maximum choice, control and power over the support services they receive.
>
> We will always fulfil our responsibility to provide care and protection for those who through their illness or disability are genuinely unable to express needs and wants or exercise control. However, the right

to self-determination will be at the heart of a reformed system only constrained by the realities of finite resources and levels of protection, which should be responsible but not risk averse.

Over time, people who use social care services and their families will increasingly shape and commission their own services. Personal Budgets will ensure people receiving public funding use available resources to choose their own support services – a right previously available only to self-funders. The state and statutory agencies will have a different not lesser role – more active and enabling, less controlling. (HM Government, 2007, p 2)

Clearly, there are cases where judgements are made to override a person's preferences. Young children's views are often overridden by parents, and some individuals may not be able to make good decisions. The Mental Capacity Act 2005 (Part 1 [2, 1]) states that 'a person lacks capacity in relation to a matter if at the material time he is unable to make a decision for himself in relation to the matter because of an impairment of, or a disturbance in the functioning of, the mind or brain'. However, even in challenging cases such as that of a person with learning disabilities, the government is keen to extend consumer sovereignty as far as possible:

Like other people, people with learning disabilities want a real say in where they live, what work they should do and who looks after them. But for too many people with learning disabilities, these are currently unattainable goals. We believe that everyone should be able to make choices. This includes people with severe and profound disabilities who, with the right help and support, can make important choices and express preferences about their day to day lives. (DH, 2001, p 24)

Although consumer sovereignty appears to be more strongly supported than ever before, there has been recent discussion of the case for more intervention in consumer choice.

Thus, behavioural economists have pointed out that people can do things that conflict with axiomatic rationality (that is, people working out all the mathematical and logical implications of a choice). People can, for example, make inconsistent choices, so that they may at times act as if they prefer A to B, but later may prefer B to A. Such preferences can be exploited in the market by a 'money-pump' approach, which charges a person exhibiting such inconsistency for exchanging A for B, then charges them for exchanging B for A. One approach to such problems is to make the value judgement that nevertheless freedom of choice is more important (Sugden, 2004) or to question whether acting in accordance with axiomatic rationality is always possible or leads to a better life (Berg and Gigerenzer, 2010).

Another approach is to examine where people may be thought to make systematic errors in their choices and seek to mitigate these errors by government intervention. This is the basis of the recent development of what has been called 'libertarian paternalism' (Sunstein and Thaler, 2003; Thaler and Sunstein, 2003) or 'asymmetric conservatism' (Camerer et al, 2003).

One of the areas where people may depart from axiomatic rationality is in choices over time. There is some evidence that people make short-sighted choices. People may, for example, be short-sighted in their approach to prevention. We have already discussed some problems with prevention above. However, an additional problem is that preventive actions often involve incurring a current cost in order to gain a future subjective benefit, and people may be short-sighted in considering these choices. Thus, the acts of saving for a pension, taking exercise, cleaning one's teeth and dieting involve incurring current costs to secure conjectured future benefits. Similarly, abstaining from a cigarette, a doughnut or alcohol involves making a current sacrifice to obtain conjectured future benefits (Thaler and Sunstein, 2008, p 73). Laibson (1997) shows how consumers suffer from excessive impulsiveness and may wish to constrain themselves to avoid the problem, while O'Donoghue and Rabin (2006) argue that consumers might want to be taxed on consumption of unhealthy foods with the proceeds returned to them.

Such arguments have led Thaler and Sunstein (2008) to suggest that the government should intervene to set 'default' options for some choices where people might be prone to such errors. For example, well-designed default pension arrangements might be set in place by the government automatically for all, and behavioural economics predicts that most would leave them in place: 'Never underestimate the power of inertia ... that power can be harnessed. If private companies or public officials think that one policy produces better outcomes, they can greatly influence the outcomes by choosing it as the default' (Thaler and Sunstein, 2008, p 8). Against the charge of authoritarianism, Thaler and Sunstein (2008) argue that these default choices should be designed to be easy for the individual to undo if they wish.

The same arguments might be used by the government to intervene in consumer choices over preventive care. Caution is needed, however, because of the possible conflict with democracy mentioned above. And as Glaeser (2006) argues, governments may also miscalculate, may take a short-term view and may have weaker incentives to get choices right than individuals. Support for this view comes from a recent evaluation of pension policy in the United Kingdom (UK):

> In the face of imperfect information and regular changes in policy, it is hard for individuals to make 'rational' choices concerning life cycle saving. In my view, it is this, rather than short-sightedness or other defects of individual planning, that lies at the heart of the 'saving problem'. The tendency has been for each successive political administration to belittle previous pension reforms and to trumpet new 'fundamental' reforms of the pension programme, often before

any such reform programme has been thought out coherently. (Disney, 2005, p 262)

So far we have looked at how commissioning could work as part of a market system of care in the case where people know what they want, or know how to buy advice on choosing what they want. We have also examined the trickier case where the market is delivering what people want, but where a case is advanced that what they want is 'wrong'. These latter arguments are hazardous, but if accepted, they suggest a case for government intervention. The argument in this latter case is that although the market is 'succeeding', it is succeeding in delivering the consumer the wrong things. A second, more straightforward case for government intervention relates to situations where preferences are not being brought into doubt, but where the market is failing to deliver in line with those preferences. Economists generally see the role of the public sector as being to correct market failure and have analysed a wide range of situations in which a market may fail[3] – and we now provide a brief review of such cases.

Market failure

Markets are considered likely to fail for a number of reasons: monopoly, externalities, public goods problems, incomplete markets and information failures, and the pattern of income distribution that results from market forces. We review these in turn.

Monopoly

The economists' optimality theorems that markets work to generate good results involve an assumption that markets are competitive. However, a local market may be too small to support competition between firms at a level of operation that allows economies of scale to be secured, so that the market becomes dominated by a small number of firms. Nevertheless, competition may still operate successfully if such markets are *contestable* (Baumol et al, 1982; Baumol and Willig, 1986). When a market is contestable, monopoly profits can be prevented if existing suppliers keep prices down because they believe they would be otherwise vulnerable to 'hit-and-run' competition from another supplier. However, if entry and exit to the market is not easy, this mechanism may not work. In these circumstances, another solution to this problem, first suggested by Demsetz (1968), is to replace competition *in* the market by competition *for* the market. Government, or local government, would thereby invite firms to tender competitively to supply all, or a large share, of local demand. The competition between firms to secure the contract would supply the competitive pressure to prevent the monopoly pricing that might otherwise obtain. Managing this process supplies a clear role for commissioning.

Externalities/public goods problems, incomplete markets and information failures

Another reason why the market may fail is as a result of externalities or public goods problems. An externality occurs when a cost or benefit of market activity is not reflected in prices. So, for example, if there was a private market for refuse collection, a resident would consider the benefit to themselves of refuse collection but perhaps not the benefit to neighbours. Similarly, a person considering whether or not to get vaccinated, or treated for an infectious disease, may not consider the benefits to others of being treated. There are also likely to be 'caring externalities' whereby people other than the person being cared for attach benefit to the provision of care (Culyer, 1989; Jacobsson et al, 2005). When there are positive externalities, the operation of the market is likely to provide too little of the service.

Relatedly, when a service has very strong externalities that apply to all in an area, the case becomes that of a local public good, and supply through the market will lead to substantial under-provision. Local public goods include the local government 'street scene', roads, local parks, criminal justice and law and order, disease prevention, substance misuse prevention and aspects of education such as citizenship. Economists generally conclude that there is therefore a role for government subsidy or finance of such services (Gruber, 2010) and managing the purchase of these services is an important role for commissioning.

Two further market failures may lead to a need for government intervention: incomplete markets and information failures (Stiglitz, 2000, pp 81-5). Because of the problems of asymmetric information outlined above, some markets may not exist. Insurance against unemployment, chronic illness and care in old age is not generally available on the market. Loans for home purchasers with a poor credit rating and for students with little collateral are also not well supplied by the market and the government may step in with finance, although this is not always without hazard, as has been found in the housing mortgage market. Lastly, markets may at times fail in the provision of information.

Distribution of income

A further argument for government intervention is that markets may operate efficiently but may lead to a distribution of income that voters may wish to change. This argument is related to the 'caring externalities' argument noted above. Private charity may provide an important channel of redistribution, but beyond this, further redistribution may be enforced using the government's power to tax.

If the purpose of redistribution is to reduce poverty, then, given consumer sovereignty, it is a commonplace of standard economic texts to demonstrate that a transfer in kind (such as subsidised housing or free healthcare) will usually confer less benefit on the recipient than receipt of the cash cost of the benefit (Rosen, 2005, pp 158-9; see also Friedman, 1962, chapter 7, and Peacock and Berry, 1951). The intuition behind this argument is that cash allows the recipient more freedom to spend on their highest priorities than receipt of a benefit in kind (which they may not have seen as a high priority). For example, a person given better housing may have preferred to receive the cash equivalent and spend it on food. Realisation that this is the case may explain the growing move towards personalisation and direct payments for social care, and there is evidence that such policies are preferred (Glasby and Littlechild, 2009; see also Chapter Eleven, this volume). However, if the purpose of redistribution is to make the voter-taxpayer paying for the redistribution happy, then if providing an in-kind benefit such as free healthcare rather than cash makes voters happier, this will be what politicians arrange (Pauly, 1970). Tobin (1970) argues that people may care particularly about inequality in access to certain goods and services such as healthcare and education – specific egalitarianism – and be more concerned to reduce inequality under these headings rather than provide cash to reduce inequality in a more general sense.

Having discussed the economics of commissioning in relation to the consumer or user of services, we now turn to the role of the commissioner in relation to the supplier of services. In relation to the supplier, commissioners make strategic make-or-buy decisions and also have a role in contractual relations. We discuss these in turn.

Commissioning and suppliers of services

A broad question for public organisations that can be looked at strategically and also at a more detailed level is whether they should make services or buy them. Equivalently, we may ask whether a service should be outsourced or produced by an in-house unit. Chris Lonsdale considered this question at length in Chapter Four, so here we will restrict discussion to providing a brief sketch of the economics that relate to this issue.

Since the time of Adam Smith it has been recognised that trade and specialisation provide a powerful way of improving productivity. Instead of producing something in-house with a small production run and lack of expertise, an organisation can buy from a specialist provider who can supply expertise and economies of scale by providing the service for many buyers. With such advantages, the question of whether to outsource turns to why any organisation should produce anything in-house (Coase, 1937). We examine this question below. The broad answer is that where the 'transactions costs' of using the market are high, in-house production may be preferred.

A powerful way of looking at such questions of how to organise production has recently been provided by principal-agent theory – already introduced above in relation to consumer decision making. Principal-agent theory looks at the problem a principal may encounter in getting an agent to provide goods or services. The interests of the principal and agent differ in that the principal will be seeking to minimise the cost of the desired outcome, whereas the agent will be seeking to maximise the payment for the services they provide.

The make-or-buy decision for the principal consists of deciding whether to use an in-house unit as an agent or to use an external firm. As a broad distinction, the in-house unit can be seen as being paid for its input time, whereas external contractors are more likely to be paid for the results they achieve.[4] The problem with using an in-house unit is that it may achieve inadequate results for the time it spends and thereby provide poor VFM. Hennart (1993) describes this as 'shirking', and contrasts in-house shirking with the danger of 'cheating' by the external contractor. The principal is exposed to cheating by external providers because of contractual difficulties in defining and measuring the results expected, as highlighted by transaction cost economics. Such problems include the costs of bargaining before the agreement is made and the costs of monitoring and enforcing the agreement afterwards (Gibbons, 2010; Williamson, 2010). Such specification and monitoring difficulties may allow a degree of cheating by the contractor, leading to poor VFM. If the commissioner responds to suspected cheating by making difficulties over payment, relations are likely to become adversarial. Transactions cost theory argues that, in circumstances where it is difficult to control an external contractor because of weaknesses in contracting, it may be preferable to exert the control by internal hierarchical methods through telling salaried employees what to do.

An important problem with managing by contract is that contracts will generally be incomplete, because working out what to do about all contingencies will be too costly[5] (Simon, 1955; Tirole, 2009). As Williamson (1985, p 20) argues, 'rather therefore than contemplate all conceivable bridge crossings in advance, which is a very ambitious undertaking, only bridge-crossing choices are addressed as the events unfold'. In addition, one of the parties to the contract may wish to keep their private information about likely add-ons under a shroud (Gabaix and Laibson, 2006). Reasons for a supplier wanting to keep some information to themselves relates to W. C. Fields' principle of 'never give a sucker an even break' (ODQ, 1996, p 282). Thus, a supplier may bid a low price for service A under competitive pressure in order to win the contract, knowing that if they win they will very likely be asked for a necessary add-on B, which they charge a monopoly price for to recoup their earlier under-pricing. This problem arises when one-to-many competitive bidding undergoes a 'fundamental transformation' to one-to-one bargaining when the successful contractor is appointed (Williamson, 1985, pp 61-3).

One way for the commissioner to police such problems is to respond by switching to a new supplier, but this option is not always available. For instance, it is often difficult to exit from using an existing supplier in social care because of the damage this may inflict on vulnerable service users. Switching suppliers also becomes too costly if supplying the service involves investment in relationship-specific assets by the agent and/or the principal. For example, supplying a service to a local authority may involve investment in learning about the local authority's ways of working and might involve the purchase of equipment specific to the task with little value for other uses. It might seem that the need for a supplier to make relationship-specific investments would give the commissioning body a bargaining advantage. However, contractors will be aware of this, and for this reason will only agree to tender for long-term contracts. The presence of asset specificity (Milgrom and Roberts, 1992, p 135) therefore implies that suppliers will require a long-term contract to induce them to take the relationship-related risk that such investments involve.

Although suppliers will require a long-term contract in such cases in order to induce them to tender, long-term contracts, as noted, are likely to be incomplete. A long-term relationship lacking clauses to cover all contingencies (as will be the case in all but the simplest of cases) is called a relational contract (Macneil, 1974, 1978). In such circumstances, the:

> major importance of [a] legal contract is to provide ... a framework which almost never accurately indicates real working relations, but which affords a rough indication around which such relations vary, an occasional guide in cases of doubt, and a norm of ultimate appeal when the relations cease in fact to work. (Llewellyn, 1931, pp 736-7, cited in Williamson, 2010, p 679)

In relational contracting, therefore, the parties may find it fruitful to treat the contract as a reference point (Hart and Moore, 2008). There will be occasions when the commissioner has the supplier 'over a barrel' because it may be excessively costly to stick to the letter of the contract, but later the boot may be on the other foot, and an investment in forbearance by both parties is likely to be in each other's interest (Watt, 1998, p 196). In this view, relational contracting can be seen as a repeated game, where the gains to breaching trust to capture a short-term pay off can be dwarfed by the longer-term costs generated by loss of trust (Watt, 2005). It may therefore be in the interests of both the commissioner and the supplier of services to try to train the other to behave cooperatively (Axelrod, 1984).

Conclusions

This chapter has provided a brief introduction to some of the economic issues that arise in commissioning. Economic issues arise in both the production and consumption sides of commissioning. On the *consumer* side, it is important to be clear whether consumer sovereignty does or does not apply, although this is a complex question as the discussion above shows. If consumer sovereignty applies, there may still be a role for commissioning, although it needs to be cost-effective. Where consumer sovereignty does not apply there is a more straightforward role for commissioning, although current policy is seeking to extend the application of consumer sovereignty to difficult cases. There are also market failure arguments for commissioning where the commissioning role is to attempt to correct such failures. On the *production* side, commissioners will make a key contribution to strategic make-or-buy decisions, as well as taking a long-term perspective on managing tendering, monitoring and contractual relations.

Notes

[1] Buying on someone's behalf can be quite inefficient. Waldfogel (1993, p 1328) finds that, compared with receiving the cash cost, 'gift-giving destroys between 10 per cent and a third of the value of gifts'.

[2] The Office of Fair Trading (2010, p 39) uses the term 'intermediation'; other terms used include 'person-centred planning facilitator', 'care broker', 'care navigator' (DH, 2005) and 'support broker' (Dowson and Greig, 2009).

[3] Note that 'market failure' implies no necessary conclusion of 'government success' (Stigler, 1988, pp148-9).

[4] This formulation is similar to that of Levin and Tadelis (2010).

[5] NHS Standard Contracts can be extremely lengthy and may provide an illustration of this point.

Further reading

A clear account of the market and market failure arguments for state intervention can be found in a number of texts, including:

- Bailey, S. J. (1999) *Local government economics: principles and practice*, Basingstoke: Palgrave Macmillan.
- Barr, N. (2004) *The economics of the welfare state* (4th edition), Oxford: Oxford University Press.
- Smith, S., Le Grand, J. and Propper, C. (2008) *The economics of social problems* (4th edition), Basingstoke: Palgrave Macmillan.
- Stiglitz, J. E. (2000) *Economics of the public sector* (3rd edition), New York, NY: Norton.

A useful reference on make-or-buy decisions and transactions cost economics is provided by:

- Williamson, O. E. (1996) 'Economics and organisation: a primer', *California Management Review*, vol 38, no 2, pp 131-46.

A clear account of issues relevant to the production side of commissioning can be found in:

- Douma, S. and Schreuder, H. (2008) *Economic approaches to organisations* (4th edition), London: Prentice Hall.

Useful websites

- The Library of Economics and Liberty is a useful website that explains a wide range of economic concepts and theories. It has a more pro-market point of view than some readers may prefer: www.econlib.org/
- For information on the implications of individual budgets, see www.in-control. org.uk/ and www.centreforwelfarereform.org/ (see also Chapter Eleven, this volume). A particularly helpful report on the 'economics of self-directed support' is available at www.in-control.org.uk/media/55944/in%20control%20 second%20phase%20report%20.pdf
- For more general insights into commissioning, see the NHS Information Centre: www.ic.nhs.uk/commissioning/

Reflective exercises

1. What cases can you identify of individuals where it is justifiable to overrule their market choices? Very young children present a clear case – what other cases would you include and where would you draw the line?
2. Which public services are reasonably easy for users to judge and which services involve a need for more expert judgement to be exercised?
3. Think about a service you have recently commissioned (or have read about). Where did the power lie in the relationship between commissioner and provider, and what mechanisms were available if things went wrong?
4. How can commissioners encourage the development of trust with contractors?

References

Arrow, K. J. and Debreu, G. (1954) 'The existence of an equilibrium for a competitive economy', *Econometrica*, vol XXII, pp 265-90.

Axelrod, R. (1984) *The evolution of cooperation*, New York, NY: Basic Books.

Baumol, W. J. and Willig, R. D. (1986) 'Contestability: developments since the book', *Oxford Economic Papers*, vol 38, supplement, November, pp 9-36.

Baumol, W. J., Panzar, J. C. and Willig, R. D. (1982) *Contestable markets and the theory of industry structure*, New York, NY: Harcourt Brace Jovanovich.

Benjamin, A. E. and Fennell, M. L. (2007) 'Putting the consumer first: an introduction and overview', *Health Services Research*, vol 42, no 1, part II, pp 353-61.

Berg, N. and Gigerenzer, G. (2010) 'As-if behavioral economics: neoclassical economics in disguise?', *History of Economic Ideas*, vol xviii, no 1, pp 133-65.

Camerer, C., Issacharoff, S., Loewenstein, G., O'Donoghue, T. and Rabin, M. (2003) 'Regulation for conservatives: behavioral economics and the case for asymmetric paternalism', *University of Pennsylvania Law Review*, vol 151, no 3, pp 1211-54.

Churchill, W. (1947) Speech, *The official report*, House of Commons (5th series), 11 November, vol 444, cc 206-07.

Coase, R. (1937) 'The nature of the firm', *Economica*, vol 4, pp 233-61.

Culyer, A. J. (1989) 'The normative economics of health care finance and provision', *Oxford Review of Economic Policy*, vol 5, no 1, pp 34-58.

Darby, M. R. and Karni, E. (1973) 'Free competition and the optimal amount of fraud', *Journal of Law and Economics*, vol 16, pp 67-88.

De Jaegher, K. (2010) 'Physician incentives: cure versus prevention', *Journal of Health Economics*, vol 29, pp 124-36.

Demsetz, H. (1968) 'Why regulate utilities?', *Journal of Law and Economics*, vol 11, no 1, pp 55-65.

DH (Department of Health) (2001) *Valuing people: a new strategy for learning disability for the 21st century*, London: DH.

DH (2005) *Independence, well-being and choice: our vision for the future for social care for adults in England*, London: DH.

Disney, R. (2005) 'The United Kingdom's pension programme: structure, problems and reforms', *Intereconomics*, September/October, pp 257-62.

Dowson, S. and Greig, R. (2009) 'The emergence of the independent support broker role', *Journal of Integrated Care*, vol 17, no 4, pp 22-30.

Duffy, S. and Fulton, K. (2009) *Should we ban brokerage?*, Sheffield: Centre for Welfare Reform.

Dulleck, U. and Kerschbamer, R. (2006) 'On doctors, mechanics and computer specialists: the economics of credence goods', *Journal of Economic Perspectives*, vol XLIV, March, pp 5-42.

Evans, R. G. (1974) 'Supplier-induced demand – some empirical evidence and implications', in M. Perlman (ed) *The economics of health and medical care*, London: Macmillan.

Evans, R. G. (1976) 'Modelling the objectives of the physician', in R. D. Fraser (ed) *Health economics symposium*, Kingston: Queen's University Industrial Relations Centre.

Friedman, M. (1962) *Capitalism and freedom*, Chicago, IL: University of Chicago Press.

Friedman, M. and Friedman, R. (1980) *Free to choose*, London: Secker and Warburg.

Gabaix, X. and Laibson, D. (2006) 'Shrouded attributes, consumer myopia, and information suppression in competitive markets', *Quarterly Journal of Economics*, vol 121, no 2, pp 505-39.

Gibbons, R. (2010) 'Transactions cost economics: past, present and future?', *Scandinavian Journal of Economics*, vol 122, no 2, pp 263-88.

Glaeser, E. L. (2006) 'Paternalism and psychology', *University of Chicago Law Review*, vol 73, pp 133-56.

Glasby, J. and Littlechild, R. (2009) *Direct payments and personal budgets* (2nd edition), Bristol: The Policy Press.

Glasby, J., Le Grand, J. and Duffy, S. (2009) 'A healthy choice? Direct payments and healthcare in the English NHS', *Policy & Politics*, vol 37, no 4, pp 481-97.

Gruber, J. (2010) *Public finance and public policy*, New York, NY: Worth.

Hart, O. and Moore, J. (2008) 'Contracts as reference points', *Quarterly Journal of Economics*, vol CXXII, no 1, pp 1-47.

Hennart, J.-F. (1993) 'Explaining the swollen middle: why most transactions are a mix of "market" and "hierarchy"', *Organization Science*, vol 4, no 4, pp 529-47.

HM Government (2007) *Putting People First: a shared vision and commitment to the transformation of adult social care*, London: DH.

House of Commons Health Committee (2010) *Commissioning*, Fourth Report of Session 2009-10, vol 1, London: TSO.

Jacobsson, F., Carstensen, J. and Borgquist, L. (2005) 'Caring externalities in health economic evaluation: how are they related to severity of illness?', *Health Policy*, vol 73, pp 172-82.

Jay, D. (1937) *The socialist case,* London: Faber and Faber.

Jensen, M. and Meckling, W. (1976) 'Theory of the firm: managerial behaviour, agency costs and capital structure', *Journal of Financial Economics*, vol 3, no 4, pp 305-60.

Laibson, D. (1997) 'Golden eggs and hyperbolic discounting', *Quarterly Journal of Economics*, vol 112, no 2, pp 443-477.

Lerner, A. P. (1972) 'The economics and politics of consumer sovereignty', *American Economic Review*, vol 62, no 2, pp 258-66.

Levin, J. and Tadelis, S. (2010) 'Contracting for government services: theory and evidence from US cities', *Journal of Industrial Economics*, vol LVII, September, pp 507-41.

Llewellyn, K. N. (1931) 'What price contract? An essay in perspective', *Yale Law Journal*, vol 40, no 5, pp 704-51.

Macneil, I. (1974) 'Contracts: adjustments of long-term economic relations under classical, neoclassical and relational contract law', *Northwestern University Law Review*, vol LCCII, pp 854-906.

Macneil, I. (1978) 'The many futures of contracts', *Southern California Law Review*, vol 47, no 3, pp 691-816.

Milgrom, P. and Roberts, J. (1992) *Economics, organisation and management*, Upper Saddle River, NJ: Prentice Hall.

Musgrave, R. A. (1959) *The theory of public finance*, New York, NY: McGraw-Hill.

Musgrave, R. A. and Musgrave, P. B. (1989) *Public finance in theory and practice*, New York, NY: McGraw Hill.

O'Donoghue, T. and Rabin, M. (2006) 'Optimal sin taxes', *Journal of Public Economics*, vol 90, pp 1825-49.

ODQ (1996) *Oxford dictionary of quotations*, Revised Fourth Edition, Oxford: Oxford University Press.

Office of Fair Trading (2010) *Choice and competition in public services: A guide for policy makers*, London: Office of Fair Trading and Frontier Economics, March.

Pauly, M. (1970) 'Efficiency in the provision of consumption subsidies', *Kyklos*, vol 23 pp 33-57.

Peacock, A. T. and Berry, D. (1951) 'A note on the theory of income redistribution', *Economica*, vol 18, no 69, pp 83-90.

Persky, J. (1993) 'Retrospectives: consumer sovereignty', *Journal of Economic Perspectives*, vol 7, no 1, pp 183-91.

Rosen, H. (2005) *Public finance* (7th edition), New York, NY: McGraw-Hill.

Ross, S. (1973) 'The economic theory of agency: the principal's problem', *American Economic Review*, vol 48, pp 134-9.

Sappington, D. (1991) 'Incentives in principal agent relationships', *Journal of Economic Perspectives*, vol 3, no 2, pp 45-66.

Shaw, G. B. (1930 [1906]) *The doctor's dilemma*, London: Constable & Co.

Simon, H. A. (1955) 'A behavioral model of rational choice', *Quarterly Journal of Economics*, vol 69, pp 99-118.

Smith, A. (1937 [1776]) *The wealth of nations*, New York, NY: Modern Library.

Smith, P.C., Stepan, A., Valdmanis, V. and Verheyen, P. (1997) 'Principal-agent problems in health care systems: an international perspective, *Health Policy*, vol 41, pp 37-60.

Stewart, J. and Walsh, K. (1992) 'Change in the management of public services', *Public Administration*, vol 70, pp 499-518.

Stigler, G.J. (1988) *Memoirs of an unregulated economist*, New York, NY: Basic Books.

Stiglitz, J. E. (2000) *Economics of the public sector* (3rd edition), New York, NY: Norton.

Stinchcombe, A. L. (1984) 'Third party buying: the trend and the consequences', *Social Forces*, vol 62, no 4, pp 861-83.

Sugden, R. (2004) 'The opportunity criterion: consumer sovereignty without the assumption of coherent preferences', *American Economic Review*, vol 94, no 4, pp 1014-33.

Sunstein, C. and Thaler, R. (2003) 'Libertarian paternalism is not an oxymoron', *University of Chicago Law Review*, vol 70, no 4, pp 1159-202.

Thaler, R. H. and Sunstein, C. R. (2003) 'Libertarian paternalism', *American Economic Review*, vol 93, no 2, pp 175-9.

Thaler, R. H. and Sunstein, C. R. (2008) *Nudge: improving decisions about health, wealth and happiness*, New Haven, CT, and London: Yale University Press.

Tirole, J. (2009) 'Cognition and incomplete contracts', *American Economic Review*, vol 99, no 1, pp 265-94.

Tobin, J. (1970) 'On limiting the domain of inequality', *Journal of Law and Economics*, vol 13, pp 263-77.

Toye, R. (2002) 'The "gentleman in Whitehall" reconsidered: the evolution of Douglas Jay's views on economic planning and consumer choice, 1937-1947', *Labour History Review*, vol 67, pp 187-204.

Waldfogel, J. (1993) 'The deadweight loss of Christmas', *American Economic Review*, vol 83, no 3, pp 1328-36.

Watt, P. A. (1998) 'White collar services in local government: competition and trust', in A. Coulson (ed) *Trust and contracts: relationships in local government, health and public services*, Bristol: The Policy Press.

Watt, P.A. (2005) 'Information, cooperation and trust in strategic service delivery partnerships', *Public Policy & Administration*, vol 20, no 3, pp 108-25.

Williamson, O. E. (1975) *Markets and hierarchies: analysis and antitrust implications*, New York, NY: The Free Press.

Williamson, O. E. (1985) *The economic institutions of capitalism*, New York, NY: The Free Press.

Williamson, O. E. (2010) 'Transaction cost economics: the natural progression', *American Economic Review*, vol 100, no 3, pp 673-90.

NINE

Public and user involvement in commissioning

Jo Ellins

Summary

This chapter explores:
* rationales for involving patients and the public in planning, developing and improving health and social services;
* different approaches to involvement;
* barriers to effective involvement;
* possible ways forward and signs of progress.

In recent years, patients and the public have been increasingly invited to contribute to the planning, development and improvement of health and social services. In England, the creation of a National Health Service (NHS) system for patient and public involvement (PPI) can be traced as far back as 1974 and the establishment of community health councils. But arguably the defining moment of this history was in 2001, when a statutory duty was placed on NHS organisations to 'involve and consult' their local communities in decisions about how services are run. While these developments focus on a range of different types of involvement, recent years have also seen growing interest in PPI in the commissioning cycle – and this chapter seeks to combine a more general discussion of involvement per se with more detailed analysis of involvement in commissioning.

Broadly, three different rationales have been put forward for PPI. The first of these offers a rights-based perspective. It holds that giving people a say in the services they use fosters, and is an expression of, autonomy and self-determination. This is captured by the slogan 'nothing about me, without me', which has been used by, among others, people with learning disabilities and people with mental health problems to challenge professional paternalism and push for more inclusive ways of working. For these groups, the recognition that an individual is capable of participating in their services sees the person in 'the patient' and is an essential step away from dependence and towards empowerment. On this basis, involvement is considered to be intrinsically important, a worthwhile end in itself. Historically, this is a perspective that has perhaps been more common in social care than in some areas of healthcare.

Alternatively, involvement can be seen in instrumentalist terms as a means to better ends and it is this rationale that has principally underpinned the promotion of PPI in NHS policy making. In this sense, involvement is considered an important mechanism by which the design and delivery of services can be informed by an understanding of the priorities, needs and experiences of the people who use them. The aim is to bring about health and social care that is more accessible, targeted and responsive, with the hope that this will lead to improved patient experience and outcomes. In some cases, involvement has been presented as an essential strategy for service reform and modernisation (DH, 2000).

The final rationale takes a broader view, and is most commonly used as a justification for involvement in public services more generally than in either health or social services specifically. This takes as its starting point the decline in traditional forms of political participation, as evidenced by long-term decreases in trades union and party membership and in voter turnout in local and general elections. In this context, involvement fulfils an important social function by creating new opportunities for active citizenship that have the potential to reconnect people with each other and to the public realm. Strengthening communities, reducing social exclusion and reinvigorating democracy have all been posited as desirable outcomes from this process (Stoker, 2006).

The way in which involvement is justified has important implications, above all for the criteria against which success is judged. Within a rights-based model, the availability of opportunities for people to discuss issues and share their views and experiences is paramount. Where involvement is seen as a way of achieving specific objectives, effectiveness will be measured by the outcomes that those opportunities produce. The key question guiding this measurement is whether involvement has had an impact: either on the quality and availability of local services (rationale 2), or on social and community life (rationale 3). Of course, these different rationales and the evaluation criteria that they give rise to are not mutually exclusive, may be combined and frequently overlap in policy and practice.

Against the context of these different rationales, this chapter will:

- trace the conceptual and policy development of PPI in health and social care;
- provide a critical overview of methods, considering in particular the factors that shape the success of involvement processes;
- review the evidence on the impact of involving patients and the public in the planning, development and evaluation of health and social services;
- explore the barriers and challenges to opening up decision-making processes to greater user and public influence.

While the chapter will principally focus on the NHS and adult social care in England, it will draw on a range of models, experience and examples where possible to illustrate broader themes and developments.

Patient and public involvement – concepts and policies

What is involvement?

Efforts to define the concept of 'PPI' are longstanding and ongoing. Two of the earliest contributions to these conceptual debates – from economist Albert Hirschman and public policy analyst Sherry Arnstein – continue to be influential to the present day. In *Exit, Voice and Loyalty*, Hirschman (1970) proposed that dissatisfied customers had three potential responses available to them:

- *exit*: they can withdraw from that good or service and look for a better alternative;
- *voice*: they can seek to exert pressure on the organisation concerned by communicating their dissatisfaction or offering suggestions for improvement; or
- *loyalty*: they can do nothing.

In so doing, he drew a basic distinction between a consumerist model of involvement, which requires competing providers and consumer choice (exit), and a participatory one, which is more closely aligned with the principles of citizenship and democracy (voice). To Hirschman's original framework, the World Health Organization (2005) added an additional category of 'representation'. This was intended to capture the formalised roles that patients and the public play in the governance of health services, contrasted with mechanisms for gathering public views and preferences that were described by the World Health Organization as 'voice'.

Arnstein (1969) understood involvement in terms of the relationship between citizens and officials, and the balance of power across these two groups. This was graphically represented using the image of a ladder, with eight levels of participation ranked according to the degree of control that citizens have over decisions and resources (Figure 9.1). Implicit in Arnstein's model is a normative assumption that citizens should be aiming to climb the ladder, away from bottom rungs of 'manipulation' and 'placation' by public agencies, to full 'citizen control' at the top. This is reflected in the description of the activities forming the lower rungs of the ladder as 'non-participation' and 'tokenism'. Over 40 years after it was first introduced, Arnstein's ladder model is arguably still the most influential model of participation, used by policy makers and practitioners alike. It has not, however, been without its criticisms. Tritter and McCallum (2006) argue that Arnstein's hierarchy of approaches conflates the means and ends of involvement. Therefore, certain approaches are more highly valued irrespective of whether they are appropriate to the context in which they are being applied or to the users who participate. Furthermore, they note that the model fails to take into account the depth or comprehensiveness of involvement, so does not consider the issue of *who* participates. Citizen control may not be advantageous where that control is exercised by one group of people, to the exclusion of others.

Figure 9.1: Ladder model of public participation

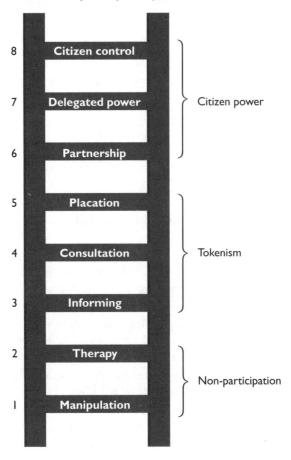

Source: Arnstein (1969)

To this I would add a further concern, which is about whether it is involvement as a *transfer of power*, or involvement as a *sharing of power*, which is likely to achieve the best outcomes for patients and the public. Health and social care organisations have much to benefit from gaining a better understanding of the needs and experiences of those who use their services. Indeed, opportunities for managers and professionals to hear and learn from patients' experiences are identified as having a key role to play in bringing about more user-centred cultures and ways of working (Crawford et al, 2004). This suggests that the greatest impact may be achieved by fostering dialogue and collaboration between service providers and users, for example by creating opportunities for partnership working. The risk of citizen control is that it transfers services from statutory authorities to citizens, but leaves the relationship between these groups unchanged.

Several of the shortcomings that arise from a linear and hierarchical conception of involvement are overcome in the approach proposed by Rowe and Frewer

(2005). They differentiate three levels of involvement, which are defined by the way in which information flows between public agencies and members of the public (see Box 9.1). The provision of information by agencies to the public is described as 'communication'. When information flows in the opposite direction – from public to agency – this is 'consultation'. In the final level there is a two-way exchange of information, a dialogue between these groups; this is termed 'participation'. While Rowe and Frewer endeavour to distinguish these levels from one another, they do not do so in a way that makes judgements about their relative merits. This is important inasmuch as it allows for recognition of the important role that information and consultation can play. Patients frequently report the need for information and providing information about local services plays a vital role in supporting choices and securing public accountability (DH, 2004). Moreover, it avoids the risk posed by Arnstein's model that certain types of involvement could be considered necessarily better irrespective of how widely they engage or what they achieve.

Box 9.1: Typology of public involvement

Communication: Information is conveyed from the public agency to members of the public. The flow of information is one way, and no response from recipients is required or sought.

Flow of information

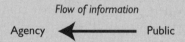

Agency → Public

Consultation: Information is conveyed by members of the public, following a process that is initiated by the agency. Typically it is the public's opinions on a specific issue or topic that are being elicited.

Flow of information

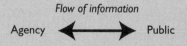

Agency ← Public

Participation: Information is exchanged between members of the public and the agency concerned. Some degree of dialogue and negotiation takes place, which may serve to transform the opinions of members of both parties.

Flow of information

Agency ←→ Public

Source: Rowe and Frewer (2005)

Recent policy context

A formal mechanism for representing public views within the NHS has been in place since the creation of community health councils in 1974. However, it was not until over 20 years later that PPI emerged as a major goal of health policy (Baggott, 2005). Soon after coming to power in 1997, the New Labour government set out its vision for the health service with a commitment 'to rebuild public confidence in the NHS as a public service, accountable to patients, open to the public and shaped by their views (DH, 1997, p 11). By the early 2000s, an infrastructure for PPI was being put in place across England, with every NHS organisation required to:

- develop a Patient Advocacy and Liaison Service (PALS);
- establish a forum through which patients and members of the public could input into the development and delivery of services;
- carry out an annual survey of patients' experiences of care.

This commitment was given a legislative basis in 2001, when a statutory duty was placed on all NHS organisations to involve and consult their local communities in developing and making changes to health services.

Legal and policy mandates for involvement are also a longstanding feature of social care. Indeed, they can be traced much further back than in healthcare – to the National Health Service and Community Care Act 1990, which made numerous references to the need to inform, consult and involve people who use services. In contrast to the NHS, a more person-centred model of involvement has sometimes emerged in social care, drawing on traditional social work principles of respect for individuals and self-determination (Kemshall and Littlechild, 2000). Social care providers have been urged to promote independence, well-being and choice, giving people greater control over their lives and over the services they use. The 2005 government Green Paper *Independence, well-being and choice* (DH, 2005, p 28) called for '[the] move from a system where people have to take what is offered to one where people have greater control over identifying the type of support or help they want, and more choice about and influence over the services on offer'. This more person-centred perspective is also reflected in the development of commissioning within social care, where service users are now being given the means to act as micro-commissioners of their own care and support (see Chapter Eleven, this volume). While the allocation of resources continues to be based on a formal needs assessment process, the development of personal budgets and direct payments potentially gives individuals much greater control over decisions about how their assessed needs are best met.

A key theme in the development of PPI within the NHS has been that of local accountability. Established as a centrally controlled service and traditionally managed through a command-and-control structure, the NHS has been subject to claims that it suffers from a 'democratic deficit' and a lack of accountability to patients and the public (see, for example, Thorlby, 2008). Efforts to devolve power are ongoing and have taken various forms. Steps have been taken to reduce the number of centralised targets, with the intention of giving NHS organisations greater flexibility to develop local plans and respond to locally defined needs and priorities. New models of local social ownership have also been promoted, including NHS foundation trusts, social enterprises and community mutuals. These models are underpinned by more inclusive and participatory governance arrangements, which have created opportunities for service users and community members to become involved in the running of NHS organisations. However, to date the pace of decentralisation has been slow and commentators have questioned whether any real devolution of power from central government to localities has taken place (Lewis and Hinton, 2008).

For some commentators (eg Fotaki et al, 2005; Greener, 2008), the recent history of PPI in the NHS can be characterised as a struggle between Hirschman's 'choice' and 'voice' models. Their analysis rests on the premise that patient choice promotes an individualistic ethic in healthcare and that this emphasises the self-interested pursuit of personal goals above all else. This is seen to be at odds with the egalitarian values on which the NHS was founded, as well as potentially diminishing interest in and the influence of approaches that seek to bring about change through collective action. Whether or not this argument is borne out over time, the rise of patient choice within virtually all sectors of the NHS is indisputable. Patients are being re-cast as 'consumers', and the range of providers from which they can choose is growing as non-NHS organisations – including those from the commercial and voluntary sectors – are being encouraged to deliver services. At the same time, efforts have been made to increase the amount of publicly available information on service quality and outcomes to inform patients' decision making. This includes initiatives such as the national NHS Choices website (www.nhs. uk), through which the public can find and compare providers using a range of indicators, including patient-reported satisfaction.

Commissioners too are expected to engage patients and the public in their work. An 'engagement cycle' has been developed to support commissioners, reflecting the opportunities for local views to influence every stage of the process from understanding needs to assessing provider performance (InHealth Associates and DH, 2009) (see Figure 9.2). The need for organisations to systematically gather and use information about what matters to patients (customer insight) and to develop an organisational infrastructure that embeds PPI into everyday working (engagement culture and systems) is emphasised. With the current financial downturn and cutting of public sector budgets, services will have to make difficult decisions about their priorities and how increasingly restricted funds are allocated. Priority setting is one area where PPI might be expected to increase within the NHS and, perhaps to a lesser extent, social care. Inviting local communities to contribute to debates about resource allocation may be necessary to ensure the perceived legitimacy of decisions that, especially where services will have to be cut, may be both sensitive and contentious (see also Chapter Three, this volume, and Williams et al, 2011).

Figure 9.2: The engagement cycle

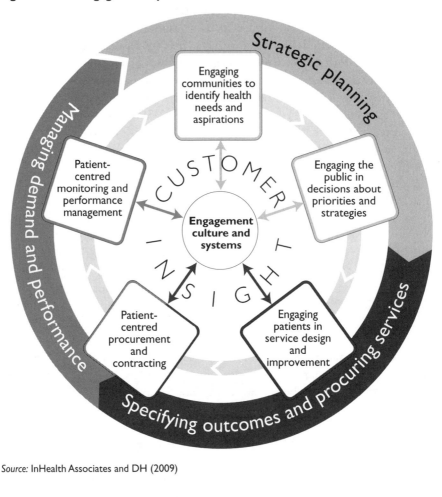

Source: InHealth Associates and DH (2009)

Methods of involvement

Types of methods

Health and social care commissioners seeking to involve patients and the public have a vast, and ever-increasing, number of methods at their disposal. Rowe and Frewer (2005) identified over 100 different mechanisms for enabling involvement – a list that, the authors themselves point out, is by no means exhaustive. These methods embody different principles and purposes, and originate from fields as diverse as community empowerment, international development, local government, organisational development and market research. The use of information and communication technologies – including interactive tools such as social networking sites, electronic feedback systems and online discussion forums – is opening up new ways for organisations to interact with and gather information from the public, leading to the rise of what has been termed 'e-participation'. In particular, these tools are being used to target groups for whom traditional approaches to involvement such as public meetings are likely to be less appealing or convenient, including young people and working adults.

Among this array of tools and techniques, there is no one method of involvement that is most suitable and effective in all situations. This is because involvement methods vary across a number of factors: the purpose they were developed for, the way they compose the process, the number of participants they require, the time and resources needed, the level and nature of involvement they generate and so on. On this issue, Abelson and Gauvin (2006, p 3) note, 'The search for a single "best" public participation approach that can be applied to any situation is unlikely to bear fruit but ... it is possible to identify *better* methods than others, methods that are better suited to different situations and perhaps even a "best" method for different but definable contexts.' As this suggests, the context in which a method is being used and the way it is applied are as important in determining the success of the involvement process as the method itself. Any consideration of the 'right' way to involve raises questions about the needs and interests of the particular group whose views are being sought. This brings into focus not only whether a method *encourages* participation in the sense that it is appealing to the group concerned and sustains their interest, but also whether it *enables* participation by ensuring that there are clear, accessible and appropriate ways for them to take part. One of the most common findings emerging from research in this area, which is frequently emphasised in involvement guidance and toolkits, is that 'one size doesn't fit all'.

Rowe and Frewer's typology described above provides a useful starting point for assessing and selecting involvement methods, based on whether organisations want to give information, solicit opinions or engage in a process of dialogue and negotiation. Table 9.1 gives examples of some of the most commonly used methods, separated into these three categories. Many of the consultation and feedback mechanisms found in the middle column of the table, such as surveys and opinion polls, carry the benefit that they can be used to access the views of large and representative samples of the public, for relatively low costs, using standardised tools that can be repeated many times. Their main limitation, however,

Table 9.1: Commonly used methods of involvement classified according to Rowe and Frewer's (2005) typology

Communication	Consultation	Participation
– Patient leaflets	– Patient surveys	– User representatives on
– Organisational websites	– Focus groups	committees
– Annual reports	– Patient diaries	– Partnership boards
– Newsletters	– Public consultations	– Citizens' juries
– Local press	– Complaints systems	– Deliberative polling
– Roadshows	– Comments cards	– Stakeholder conferences
– Noticeboards	– Public opinion polls	– Participatory appraisal
	– Health panels	

is that they only take a snapshot of views at a point in time, rather than providing participants with opportunities to reflect on and discuss the issues raised and – perhaps in so doing – come to a more informed view.

This makes consultation and feedback mechanisms less well suited to supporting public involvement in complex or controversial commissioning decisions, such as prioritising needs, allocating resources or redesigning services. Such decisions, as Abelson et al (2003, p 240) point out:

> require a more informed citizenry that has weighed the evidence on the issue, discussed and debated potential decision options and arrived at a mutually agreed upon decision or at least one by which all parties can abide. An active, engaged citizen (rather than the passive recipient of information) is the prescription of the day.

In response to this need for greater dialogue and discussion between stakeholders involved in decision-making processes, a number of 'deliberative' methods have emerged; examples include citizens' juries, consensus conferences and deliberative polling (see Chapter Three for more discussion of deliberative methods). The features of these methods vary, but what they share in common is a procedural approach in which participants are provided with information about the issue under consideration, given opportunities to explore that information and their views together, and then asked to make a judgement or offer recommendations (Abelson et al, 2003). Although these processes tend to encourage consensus, they can also play a role in identifying a range of values and opinions on a particular subject. Another recent innovation is experience-based design, where staff and patients work together to identify ways in which services can be redesigned to improve patients' experiences (Bate and Robert, 2006). Whereas deliberative methods may enable patients and the public to play a fuller and more informed role in decision making, especially in relation to complex issues, experience-based design goes further by seeing them as a co-producer of health outcomes.

What methods are currently used?

A 2009 survey of primary care trusts (PCTs) in England provides insight into the methods that are being used to involve patients and the public in commissioning (Picker Institute Europe, 2009). Respondents reported a wide range of approaches that had been employed in their organisations to involve local communities in the various stages of the commissioning process. These included:

- different types of events, forums and panels;
- joint working activities with other public sector agencies or voluntary sector organisations;
- technologically driven approaches;

- research and evaluation methods;
- campaigns and advertising.

Despite this evidence of diversity and creativity, the survey found that it was four more traditional methods of consultation that were most commonly – almost universally – used by PCTs:

- public meetings (used by 93% of respondents);
- formal consultation (88%);
- focus groups (87%);
- surveys (87%).

A note of concern was expressed by the authors of the survey about the limitations of these methods for engaging marginalised communities, who commented that:

> With few exceptions, the survey does not suggest that PCTs are putting resources into developing targeted approaches to engagement that are specifically designed to identify, understand and overcome the particular barriers to engagement that risk excluding 'harder to reach'/'seldom heard' groups and communities. (Picker Institute Europe, 2009, p 23)

At least in part, the popularity of methods such as surveys and focus groups reflects the broader policy context in which consultation and feedback have formed a central part of the vision for PPI in the NHS. Gathering patient feedback, in particular, has been strongly emphasised as a lever for service improvement. The mainstay of the current approach in England is a national patient survey programme, which annually measures and reports patients' experiences of care across different services and settings. This has presented a picture of what matters most to NHS patients, encompassing eight key dimensions (see Box 9.2). The survey programme has also been used to track trends in patients' experiences (Richards and Coulter, 2007). Longitudinal analysis has shown improvements in a number of areas, particularly those – such as waiting times, cancer care and coronary heart disease – that have been the subject of substantial investment and coordinated action since the early 2000s. Nonetheless, it has also identified many other aspects where patients' experiences fall short of their expectations or of expected standards of care, including:

- involvement in decision making;
- support for self care;
- provision of information;
- privacy during inpatient care;
- access to out-of-hours care.

Box 9.2: Aspects of care that NHS patients consider to be most important

- Fast access to reliable health advice.
- Effective treatment delivered by trusted professionals.
- Involvement in decisions and respect for preferences.
- Clear, comprehensible information and support for self-care.
- Attention to physical and environmental needs.
- Emotional support, empathy and respect.
- Involvement of, and support for, family and carers.
- Continuity of care and smooth transitions.

Source: Richards and Coulter (2007)

The overall conclusion that can be drawn from this research is that progress towards patient-centred care is perceptible but slow, and that paternalist approaches are still in evidence across the NHS.

Feedback systems such as the national patient survey programme in England – and similar programmes in Scotland, the United States (US) and Australia – have been specifically developed for health services to use as a tool for quality improvement. Their approach asks patients to provide factual reports on specific aspects of care, from which it may be possible to identify areas needing action or further investigation. Evidence that patient feedback is routinely being used in this way, however, is limited (Reeves and Seccombe, 2008). Research by Davies and Cleary (2005) with health professionals and managers in the US found three types of barrier to the use of patient survey data in quality improvement:

- *organisational*: including lack of supporting values for patient-centred care, lack of quality improvement infrastructure and competing priorities;
- *professional*: including clinical scepticism, defensiveness and resistance to change and lack of staff training and support;
- *data related*: including lack of timely feedback of results, felt lack of expertise with survey methods and lack of specificity in the findings.

Some of the data-related barriers identified, such as lack of timeliness and specificity, are starting to be addressed by the development of real-time technologies. These enable patients to provide feedback during or near to the point of care, at an individual ward, service or even clinician level. Nonetheless, Davies and Cleary's findings suggest that progress in developing a culture of, and systems for, quality improvement is also necessary to ensure that patient feedback is used to bring about change.

Involvement in practice: current experiences and new horizons

Current experiences

While involvement – as discussed at the beginning of this chapter – can be seen as a good in itself, organisations and commissioners investing time and resources in involvement activities and those taking part are likely to be interested in what their efforts have achieved. Indeed, helping to improve patient care, or to prevent problems that they have experienced happening to others in the future, are key motivations for people to get involved in their local health and social services (see, for example, Mauger et al, 2010). A systematic review of the evidence on involving patients in the planning and development of healthcare found that very few initiatives had evaluated the impact of this process (Crawford et al, 2004). The evidence that the review team was able to gather suggested that patients welcomed the opportunity to participate in initiatives and benefited personally in terms of improved self-esteem. A small number of examples of where involvement had led to changes in services were found, but rarely was the impact of those changes on the quality or effectiveness of services assessed. Similar conclusions have been reached by others. For example, a review of user involvement in social care commented on the lack of research and evaluation to measure impact, and the tendency for organisations to focus only on benefits to participants rather than on whether wider changes had been achieved (Carr, 2004).

Within the NHS, a national study of PPI by former regulator the Healthcare Commission reported that there were pockets of good engagement practice across the service, but little evidence that patients' views routinely or systematically influenced decision making (Healthcare Commission, 2009). It also found that patients were far more likely to have been given the opportunity to contribute to service plans and designs than to influence decisions about local priorities, the allocation of funds or the quality and safety of care. In an inquiry by the House of Commons Health Select Committee (2007, p 84), the possibility that public consultations were being carried out by NHS organisations simply to fulfil statutory requirements was raised: 'In theory there is a good system for consulting about important local proposals for change. In practice, there is much frustration and disappointment. Too often it seems to the public that decisions have been made before the consultation takes place.'

The findings of the most recent Citizenship Survey lend further support to this proposition about perceived powerlessness among the public (DCLG, 2010). Of the 10,000 people living in England and Wales who took part in the survey, little more than one third (37%) felt that they could influence decisions in their local area. Another common theme emerging from research is that the vast majority of involvement takes the form of information-gathering activities based on consultation and feedback; by contrast, approaches that promote partnership and collaboration between the providers and users of health services are used far less frequently (see, for example, Gagliardi et al, 2008).

A number of barriers to more effective involvement in health and social care have been identified. Professionals and managers generally report being supportive of the principle of user involvement. Yet in practice they have often been reluctant to share decisions with other stakeholders and have been able to use their power to limit public debate. As Crawford et al (2004) suggest, this may be symptomatic of a more deep-seated resistance to change in some organisations, than an unwillingness to engage with the needs and views of service users per se. Nonetheless, many studies have uncovered that public officials draw a distinction – sometimes explicitly, but more often implicitly – between their own 'expert knowledge' and the 'lay opinions' of patients or members of the public, which makes it difficult for the latter to have their contributions recognised and valued (see, for example, Barnes et al, 2007). This problem may be compounded by the fact that involvement is not routinely accompanied by opportunities for training and support – either to help participants develop their knowledge, confidence and skills; or for professionals to explore how and why users may be involved and reflect on their practice. Time and resource constraints present further barriers. Tight organisational timescales for decision making can effectively preclude approaches that seek to foster dialogue, negotiate outcomes and engage marginalised communities (SCIE, 2008). In such situations, a one-off consultation activity may be all that is possible. This disjuncture between the timescales for organisational decision making and those for involvement is reflected in the survey of PCT commissioners described above (Picker Institute Europe, 2009). Reported by 53% of respondents, 'difficulty ensuring that information from patient and public involvement work is available early enough in decision-making processes' was the most commonly cited barrier to more user-driven commissioning

New horizons

Both despite, and in response to, the challenges described above, efforts to improve the process and outcomes of PPI are under way. In particular, attention is shifting towards the changes that organisations need to make to become more responsive to users' needs and embed involvement in their everyday practice. Recent guidance for the NHS outlined the various steps that could be taken to build an 'involving organisation' (DH, 2008). The role that board members and senior managers should play in championing and celebrating involvement work and leading by example was highlighted. Engaging frontline staff in designing and carrying out involvement activities, as well as expecting them to act on the views expressed, was another recommendation. A similar message was conveyed by the authors of a recent national study, which explored user involvement in the commissioning of health and social services (Mauger et al, 2010, p 10):

> The concept of user involvement has been talked about, thought about and implemented in various ways by many organisations over many years. The challenge posed now is that for user involvement to

become an integral part of strategic commissioning requires a whole organisation approach and the political and cultural leadership and change that this entails.

Various guidance documents have proposed factors that are considered essential for successful user involvement – an example of these is shown in Box 9.3.

There is also growing recognition of the limitations of conventional involvement methods for engaging minority and marginalised groups such as older people, people from minority ethnic communities and people with physical and learning disabilities (SCIE, 2008). Those seeking to involve are being encouraged to identify and address the – often substantial – barriers to participation that these groups can face, which may be attitudinal, organisational, cultural and physical in kind. Ensuring that 'local voice' is not limited to groups that are well organised and articulate is particularly important at the earlier stages of the commissioning cycle, so that *all* local needs are recognised in decisions about planning and prioritising services. An approach is called for that focuses on building visibility, trust and mutual understanding *before* asking people to participate in activities or share their opinions and experiences. To this end, there is much scope for health and social care organisations to work in partnership with local voluntary sector and community groups given that they are more likely to be known and trusted by marginalised communities. One approach that is gaining popularity is user/

Box 9.3: Public and user involvement success factors

- Be clear about the aims and scope of involvement before contacting service users.
- Make the aims and scope of involvement clear to users and carers who participate.
- Ensure that your organisation is committed to acting on the views of service users before user involvement begins.
- Before embarking on new initiatives to involve service users, find out what has taken place previously.
- If possible, encourage local service users to express their aims and demands, too.
- Make sure that you allow adequate time and resources to support user involvement.
- Consider how to give feedback to service users who participate.
- Ask yourself how important it is for those service users who participate to represent users' views in general. Using a range of methods of user involvement will help you access a range of views.
- Ensure that adequate information, time, and administrative and financial support is available for service users.
- Ensure that the staff of your organisation who are involved in the process of user involvement are committed to making it a success.

Source: NHS Service Delivery and Organisation R&D Programme (2004)

---

community-led consultation or feedback. As the example in Box 9.4 illustrates, with appropriate training and support, service users are successfully leading involvement processes, and are helping health and social care organisations to reach and engage individuals whose voices might otherwise be seldom heard.

Box 9.4: Older people as researchers

Extensive consultation with members of the public and stakeholders in Coventry identified the experiences of older people in hospital and after discharge as a priority area. Following this, an 'Older Patient Experience Survey' was developed to provide insights into good and bad practices, and opportunities for improvement in the patient pathway. Thirteen older people from the local area were recruited and given training to be user researchers – they helped develop the survey tool, carried out all interviews with patients and carers (in both hospital and home settings) and participated in the analysis of the findings. The learning from a previous project that employed the user research model was that service users felt more comfortable providing feedback and could be more honest in their opinions than if the person interviewing them had been a health professional. User researchers co-presented the findings with the project team to local health and social care organisations, and contributed to monitoring the action plan that was subsequently produced to address key areas. The importance of obtaining feedback from older people was recognised by one user researcher, who commented "The patients being involved in the study felt it helped them with their stay; they felt that they were being taken notice of and that their opinions counted." Since the work on hospital stay and discharge, user researchers have led other feedback activities, including a project with service users who have physical and sensory impairments.

Source: Coventry City Council (2007)

Conclusion

This chapter has explored the issue of PPI from the perspectives of theory, policy and practice. Although different rationales are put forward for involving people in decisions about health and social care, both organisations and participants are likely to want to see improvements in services as a result of their efforts. A key component of successful involvement is the selection of a method that is engaging, enabling and appropriate – to the circumstances, the target group and the decision to be taken. But while the 'right' method can yield rich insights into the needs and experiences of people using services, it cannot of itself deliver improvements in those services. An organisational culture that values patients' experiences and an infrastructure to support quality improvement based on patients' views are equally important.

Further reading

- Department of Health (2008) *Real involvement*, London: DH, offers practical guidance on designing and carrying out involvement and using the findings to improve services. It includes sections on PPI in commissioning and contracting.
- Mauger, S., Deuchars, G., Sexton, S. and Schehrer, S. (2010) *Involving users in commissioning local services*, York: Joseph Rowntree Foundation, brings together research evidence and good practice examples to consider where and how users can be involved in commissioning services in health and social care.
- Social Care Institute for Excellence (2008) *Seldom heard: developing inclusive participation in social care*, London: SCIE, summarises the barriers to engaging minority and marginalised groups, and looks at strategies for overcoming these to develop more inclusive approaches to involvement.
- Kemshall, H. and Littlechild, R. (2000) *User involvement and participation in social care*, London: Jessica Kingsley Publishers, provides an overview of the context and rationales for user participation in social care, followed by chapters focusing on the involvement of specific user groups, including children, older people and disabled people.
- Martin, G. (2009) 'Whose health, whose care, whose say? Some comments on public involvement in new NHS commissioning arrangements, *Critical Public Health*, vol 19, pp 123-32, reports on research summarising early experiences of involving patients and the public in commissioning within the NHS.

Useful websites

- Community Development Exchange: www.cdx.org.uk/
- HealthTalk Online: www.healthtalkonline.org/
- Involve: www.involve.org.uk/
- Picker Institute Europe: www.pickereurope.org/
- Shaping Our Lives: www.shapingourlives.org.uk/

Reflective exercises

1. Using Arnstein's ladder of participation in Figure 9.1, reflect on examples of PPI from your own organisation/profession. Which rungs of the ladder are most common and are different levels of involvement appropriate for different types of issue/decision?
2. Using Rowe and Frewer's categories and typology from Box 9.1 and Table 9.1, which types of and approaches to involvement have you undertaken in your own organisation and how did you choose which approach was most appropriate?
3. Reflect on a situation where your organisation or profession wanted to seek the views of people using services. What sort of information/experience did

they wish to explore, how did they choose their approach and what impact did this have?

4. Reflecting on local involvement mechanisms, how appropriate are these to seeking a broad range of views (including groups that are seldom heard)?

References

Abelson, J. and Gauvin, F. (2006) *Assessing the impacts of public participation: concepts, evidence and policy implications*, Ottowa: Canadian Policy Research Networks.

Abelson, J., Forest, P.-G., Eyles, J., Smith, P., Martin, E. and Gauvin, F.-P. (2003) 'Deliberations about deliberative methods: issues in the design and evaluation of public participation processes', *Social Science and Medicine*, vol 57, pp 239-51.

Arnstein, S. (1969) 'A ladder of citizen participation', *Journal of the American Institute of Planners*, vol 35, no 4, pp 216-24.

Baggott, R. (2005) 'A funny thing happened on the way to the forum: the reform of patient and public involvement in England', *Public Administration*, vol 83, no 3, pp 533-51.

Barnes, M., Newman, J. and Sullivan, H. C. (2007) *Power, participation and political renewal: case studies in public participation*, Bristol: The Policy Press.

Bate, P. and Robert, G. (2006) 'Experience-based design: from redesigning the system around the patient to co-designing services with the patient', *Quality and Safety in Health Care*, vol 15, pp 307-10.

Carr, S. (2004) *Has service user participation made a difference to social care services?*, London: Social Care Institute for Excellence.

Coventry City Council (2007) *Learning from experience: older people in hospital and after discharge*, Coventry: Coventry City Council.

Crawford, M., Rutter, D. and Thelwall, S. (2004) *User involvement in change management: a review of the literature*, London: NHS SDO.

Davies, E. and Cleary, P. (2005) 'Hearing the patients' voice? Factors affecting the use of patient survey data in quality improvement', *Quality and Safety in Health Care*, vol 14, pp 428-432.

DCLG (Department for Communities and Local Government) (2010) *Citizenship survey 2009-2010*, London: DCLG.

DH (Department of Health) (1997) *The new NHS: modern, dependable*, London: DH.

DH (2000) *The NHS plan: a plan for investment, a plan for reform*, London: TSO.

DH (2004) *Better information, better choices, better health: putting information at the centre of health*, London: DH.

DH (2005) *Independence, well-being and choice*, Green Paper, Cm 6499, London: TSO.

DH (2008) *Real involvement: working with people to improve health services*, London: DH.

Fotaki, M., Boyd, A., Smith, L., McDonald, R., Roland, M., Sheaff, R., Edwards, A. and Elwyn, G. (2005) *Patient choice and the organisation and delivery of health services: scoping review*, London: NHS SDO.

Gagliardi, A., Lemieux-Charles, L., Brown, A. D., Sullivan, T. and Goel, V. (2008) 'Barriers to patient involvement in health service planning and evaluation: an exploratory study', *Patient Education and Counseling*, vol 70, pp 234-41.

Greener, I. (2008) 'Choice or voice? Introduction to the themed section', *Social Policy and Society*, vol 7, pp 197-200.

Healthcare Commission (2009) *Listening, learning, working together? A national study of how well healthcare organisations engage local people in planning and improving their services*, London: Healthcare Commission.

Hirschman, A. (1970) *Exit, voice and loyalty: responses to decline in firms, organizations and states*, Cambridge, MA: Harvard University Press.

House of Commons Health Select Committee (2007) *Patient and public involvement in the NHS: third report of session 2006-7*, London: TSO.

InHealth Associates and DH (Department of Health) (2009) *The engagement cycle: a new way of thinking about patient and public engagement (PPE) in world class commissioning*, London: DH.

Kemshall, H. and Littlechild, R. (eds) (2000) *User involvement and participation in social care: research informing practice*, London: Jessica Kingsley Publishers.

Lewis, R. and Hinton, L. (2008) 'Citizen and staff involvement in health service decision-making: have National Health Service foundation trusts in England given stakeholders a louder voice?', *Journal of Health Services Research and Policy*, vol 13, pp 19-25.

Mauger, S., Deuchars, G., Sexton, S. and Schehrer, S. (2010) *Involving users in commissioning local services*, York: Joseph Rowntree Foundation.

NHS Service Delivery and Organisation R&D Programme (2004) *How managers can help users to bring about change in the NHS (briefing paper)*, London: NHS SDO.

Picker Institute Europe (2009) *Patient and public engagement: the early impact of world class commissioning*, Oxford: Picker Institute Europe.

Reeves, R. and Seccombe, I. (2008) 'Do patient surveys work? The influence of a national survey programme on local quality-improvement initiatives', *Quality and Safety in Health Care*, vol 17, pp 437-41.

Richards, N. and Coulter, A. (2007) *Is the NHS becoming more patient-centred? Trends from the national surveys of NHS patients in England 2002-7*, Oxford: Picker Institute Europe.

Rowe, G. and Frewer, L. (2005) 'A typology of public engagement mechanisms', *Science, Technology and Human Values*, vol 30, pp 251-90.

SCIE (Social Care Institute for Excellence) (2008) *Seldom heard: developing inclusive participation in social care*, London: SCIE.

Stoker, G. (2006) *Why politics matters: making democracy work*, Basingstoke: Palgrave Macmillan.

Thorlby, R., Lewis, R. and Dixon, J. (2008) *Should primary care trusts be made more locally accountable?*, London: King's Fund.

Tritter, J. and McCallum, A. (2006) 'The snakes and ladders of user involvement: moving beyond Arnstein', *Health Policy*, vol 76, pp 156-68.

Williams, I., Robinson, S. and Dickinson, H. (2011) *Rationing in health care: the theory and practice of priority setting*, Bristol: The Policy Press.

World Health Organization (2005) *Ninth futures forum on health systems governance and public participation*, Copenhagen: WHO.

TEN

The impact of joint commissioning

Helen Dickinson and Alyson Nicholds

Summary

This chapter explores:
- the nature of joint commissioning and the claims made for its potential impact;
- a brief history of joint commissioning;
- the evidence base behind joint commissioning;
- key drivers and possible outcomes.

The need for health and social care agencies to work together has been an established part of the national policy context for at least 30 years, but this has become particularly pronounced since the late 1990s. Although health and social care agencies are essentially independent of one another, the work that these agencies does often overlaps – particularly for individuals and groups with complex or chronic needs. As such, it has long been argued that health and social care should work together in partnership (see Glasby and Dickinson, 2008, for further discussion). Indeed, it seems almost heretical to question the established notion that by working together health and social care agencies might be able to produce better services and better outcomes for service users.

At the same time that joint working has been gaining increasing interest, so too has the role of commissioning in the public sector. As chapters in this text have already demonstrated, local authorities have had a more established tradition in demand-side reforms, but since 2004 the National Health Service (NHS) has also increasingly shifted responsibility towards devolved commissioning arrangements. As commissioning has become a more important part of the health policy arena, so too has a focus on those commissioning activities that take place in conjunction with other agencies. Against this background there have been increasing references to the importance of joint commissioning in policy and practice documents (see, for example, DH, 1995, 2010a). But difficulties in defining what joint commissioning actually is and what it seeks to achieve means that it is difficult to research. Although in a broad sense the idea that health and social care agencies undertaking joint needs assessments and commissioning services might seem like it should improve outcomes for local populations, the evidence base to support this notion is limited.

This chapter reviews the evidence concerning the impacts of joint commissioning. In doing so we find that there are a number of difficulties in being definitive about the evidence base. Joint commissioning has been exhorted in a range of policies across national and local government departments, yet often with little clarity of what is meant by this concept or what it should achieve in practice. Health and social care agencies have a legal duty to undertake needs assessments for their local areas that should be used to set commissioning priorities (DH, 2007b), but beyond a general notion that working together should make services and service user outcomes better, there is little more in terms of what successful joint commissioning looks like – or the type of impacts it should produce. Part of the difficulty seems to lie in the fact that joint commissioning is, by definition, more complex than commissioning in single agency settings, and is perhaps inevitably more slippery and messy as a concept and a practice as a result.

In order to start unpacking some of this complexity, the chapter starts by setting out a brief history of joint commissioning. The next section then moves on to consider some of the definitions that have been applied to joint commissioning, arguing that one of the difficulties in being clear about its impacts is that the term has been used to refer to a number of very different organisational arrangements. The chapter then moves on to consider the evidence base for joint commissioning. Despite all the rhetoric about what joint commissioning *might* produce, there is surprisingly little evidence to support this. One of the reasons often given for this are the difficulties in evaluating joint commissioning, but we argue that these issues are not insurmountable (even if the costs of doing this are significant). There is a bias in the literature towards reporting on the processes of joint commissioning, with little consideration of the outcomes. We interrogate the literature to ascertain just what it is that joint commissioning is aiming to achieve and uncover a diverse range of drivers. Ultimately, we argue that despite political rhetoric about the importance of joint commissioning, the reality at ground level often seems to lag behind somewhat. This does not mean that we should not do joint commissioning, but we need to be clear about the activities we are undertaking when doing this in practice and the types of effects we anticipate these actions to have.

A brief history of joint commissioning

The interest in joint commissioning needs to be considered against a background of a significant and longstanding focus on the importance of inter-agency collaboration between health and social care for the health and well-being of populations. This interest is illustrated well through a relatively recent Department of Health document (DH, 2007a, p 11) that states:

> Our aspiration is for better health and increased well-being for everyone. This can only be achieved by local communities in every part of the country working together to tackle inequalities and promote equality. It also means working jointly to develop services

that are more personal to individuals and provided close to home; increasingly building on a closer integration of health, social care and other service providers, helping people to stay as healthy and as independent as possible.

The need to collaborate is not a recent fad and builds on a significant interest in joint working between health and social care that goes back to at least the establishment of the welfare state (Glasby, 2007). The Beveridge Report (Beveridge, 1942) set out five major social problems that welfare services were designed to tackle – want, disease, ignorance, squalor and idleness – often referred to as the 'five giants'. Timmins (2001) outlines the programme of reform that followed this report, which involved social security, health, education, housing and a policy of full employment – each of which was constructed to combat one of Beveridge's five giant evils. Glasby (2007) argues that although the language we use to discuss welfare services has changed somewhat in the intervening years, much of the diagnosis and the solutions set up to tackle these challenges can still be mapped across onto current services (see Table 10.1). What Glasby argues is that the advent of the welfare state saw a range of services established to deal with particular social problems – often in organisational silos – and that this pattern is still evident today. Thus, when the NHS is critiqued as being a 'sickness' service, as opposed to a 'health' service, we might remember that essentially the NHS was established initially to respond to the 'giant' of disease.

Table 10.1: UK welfare services

Beveridge's giants/social problems	Government response/service
Want	Social security
Disease	NHS
Ignorance	Education
Squalor	Housing and regeneration
Idleness	Employment and leisure

Source: From Glasby (2007, p 13)

There have been no end of policies in the United Kingdom (UK) that have sought to bring together health and social care, but essentially what is still in place today are a range of top-down bureaucratic government departments that have as their core business a focus on one of these 'giants'. Although this is a helpful way of organising complex welfare services, numerous commentators have noted its limitations (see Glasby and Dickinson, 2008, for more detail). In 1998, these were reflected in a Department of Health consultation document on future relationships between health and social care (DH, 1998). Entitled *Partnership in action*, the document proposed various ways of promoting more effective partnerships, basing these on a scathing but extremely accurate critique of single agency ways of working (DH, 1998, p 3):

> All too often when people have complex needs spanning both health and social care good quality services are sacrificed for sterile arguments about boundaries. When this happens people, often the most vulnerable in our society ... and those who care for them find themselves in the no man's land between health and social services. This is not what people want or need. It places the needs of the organisation above the needs of the people they are there to serve. It is poor organisation, poor practice, poor use of taxpayers' money – it is unacceptable.

Against this background, partnership working is no longer an option (if it ever was), but is considered a core part of public services.

In recent years there has been a significant interest in joint working as a driver of quality, efficiency and effectiveness of services. Around a similar time, commissioning has also been increasingly seen as an important lever of reform in health and social care. Since the inception of the NHS market in 1991 (DH, 1989), there has been a division within the NHS between the payers (initially referred to as 'purchasers' and now termed 'commissioners') and the providers. This, as Allen et al (2009) argue, has resulted in regular reform of the payer (or demand) side of the NHS ever since with major organisational reform taking place in (to name but a few examples) 1991, 1996, 2002, 2006 and again in 2011-12 with plans to devolve commissioning further to clinical commissioning consortia (DH, 2010a). One of the primary implications of this periodic organisational turmoil is that it makes it very difficult for NHS commissioners to survive for long enough to achieve longer-term change (Smith et al, 2004; Walshe et al, 2004). The lack of effectiveness surrounding NHS commissioning has, among other things, been due to the difficulties faced by primary care trusts (PCTs) (and their predecessors, primary care groups: PCGs) in developing and sustaining necessary relationships with partners. Joint commissioning between health and social care has been seen as one way to address this, combining the reform agendas of joint working and commissioning.

Although the terminology has changed over time, various means and mechanisms have been brought about under the guise of what we now call joint commissioning. In the 1970s, there were joint consultative committees and joint planning groups, then in the 1990s, joint commissioning was brought into the public service lexicon by the Conservative government (DH, 1995). More recently, these types of arrangements have been referred to under the guise of strategic – or place-based – commissioning. Although the need for joint commissioning has remained constant since the 1970s, the amount of interest paid to this agenda has varied over time. Joint commissioning received a degree of attention in the mid to late 1990s, but this faded away to a certain extent with the advent of PCGs and then PCTs. In the last few years, joint commissioning has arguably come to the forefront of policy again, particularly with the legal requirement that local areas produce a joint strategic needs assessment and the importance that has

———

been placed on outcomes-based commissioning (Kerslake, 2007; see also Chapter Seven, this volume).

The 2010 NHS White Paper (DH, 2010a) has since outlined new commissioning responsibilities again, but has not diluted the need for joint commissioning, with the new government arguing that '[t]he arrangements for joint planning between the NHS and social care must remain.… Joint working and commissioning between PCTs and LAs [local authorities] will be of increased importance to deliver better outcomes for patients, service users and their carers' (DH, 2010a, p 6).

Against this policy background and in a difficult financial context, joint commissioning may well become even more important in the future. Although the precise policy drivers have shifted over the years and have been called different things, a few features have remained consistent: the belief that joint commissioning is a good thing amid a lack of clarity over what it is that joint commissioning is aiming to achieve in practice. In unpacking this further, this chapter now considers what is meant by joint commissioning in more detail.

What do we mean by joint commissioning?

As we sought to illustrate in the previous section, joint commissioning emerges from a long line of policy initiatives to reduce the fragmentation that exists between health and social care agencies, ostensibly with the aim of improving quality of life for service users and carers. Despite joint commissioning being a central component of much health and social care policy, we know surprisingly little about what joint commissioning means, or indeed what it looks like in practice. Rummery and Glendinning (2000, p 18) sum this up, arguing that 'there is no universally agreed definition of joint commissioning; the term can cover a wide range of activities'. To some degree we might expect this: as other chapters in this book have demonstrated, the precise definition of commissioning is often contested (see, for example, Chapter One). Yet, the issue of definition becomes even more significant when joint commissioning brings together different agencies that might have different understandings of what is meant by this concept. Health and social care agencies might also hold fundamentally different values and beliefs in terms of the types of models of care that should underpin their activities. 'Joint' commissioning implies some sense of joint consensus in terms of concepts of outcomes and models of care, but we question the degree to which this is always achieved in practice.

One possible reason for this lack of clarity relates to the continually changing policy context that seems to conflate joint commissioning with other forms of joint working (Banks, 2002). Another may relate to joint commissioning being frequently promoted as a mechanism for achieving any number of end goals (Dowling et al, 2004). Over time these aims have ranged from attempts to improve joint working between health and social care, to achieving wider well-being for whole populations through partnerships with a range of agencies that go beyond health and social care. Consequently, Hudson (2010, p 11) argues that joint commissioning exists in a predictably 'complex, confusing and contradictory' policy landscape. As a result, it appears that joint commissioning is such 'a broad and malleable concept that it can legitimately mean different things to different people' (Hudson and Willis, 1995, cited in Greig and Poxton, 2001a, p 18). Despite having various aims and often looking quite different in practice, we still call these various manifestations of joint working 'joint commissioning'. In thinking through what joint commissioning means in more detail, we reflect here on who is involved in 'joined-up' activities.

In terms of the scope of joint commissioning arrangements, a number of different commentators have provided different frameworks for thinking about the levels at which this may operate. Greig (1997) argues that joint commissioning exists at two levels: strategic and operational. Strategic joint commissioning refers to the full integration of agencies in terms of governance processes, while operational joint commissioning relates to a partial form of integration in terms of service provision. Hudson (1999) talks about commissioning at three levels: the geographical area covering all the services in that place; the team or practice covering the commissioning of some services for certain groups; and the individual-level commissioning of services for specific service users. In contrast, the Office for Public Management (2008, p 18) suggests that 'the range of different levels of commissioning can be broadly categorised as national, regional, strategic, operational and individual'. What these different frameworks indicate is that joint commissioning might not simply happen at one level. Therefore, in thinking about the impacts and activities of joint commissioning, it is important to establish what the scale and scope of these activities are. Would we expect strategic-level joint commissioning to have the same sorts of impacts on outcomes as those activities that take place at the practice or individual level and are these driven by the same sorts of interests? We now turn to the evidence base to explore these issues in more detail.

The evidence base for joint commissioning

This section seeks to examine the evidence base underpinning joint commissioning and explores the types of impacts it has had in practice. One thing that becomes apparent when we look at this literature is that there is a distinct lack of good-quality evidence about joint commissioning. Much of the evidence is often rather faith based and does not seriously interrogate joint commissioning in any great depth. This is not a new issue:

> All these initiatives still require careful evaluation to determine whether, and which benefits claimed by primary health and social services staff are also shared by service users. Which model of joint commissioning delivers most gains for patients? How easy is it for them to find out about services? Are services better coordinated? To what extent are patients' preferences taken into account? What are the consequences

for equity and citizenship?.... it is vital that the lessons from today's experiences are taken into account. (Glendinning et al, 1998, p 124)

Although more than a decade has passed, Glendinning et al's observations about the evidence deficit still ring true. As we have already indicated, joint commissioning is often seen as difficult to achieve in practice given different financial, procedural and regulatory systems. It is also challenging to evaluate given the types of factors set out by Dickinson (2008) and summarised in Box 10.1. Given that joint commissioning is so difficult to evaluate and be definitive about, it could be the case that we have little evidence about this because it is so complex to research. Yet, many other complex social initiatives are researched where similar difficulties are encountered. Although the costs of researching joint commissioning effectively may be high, the problems may not be insurmountable. One of the major difficulties in evaluating the outcomes of joint commissioning is that we are not clear about the types of outcomes that it is trying to deliver. The remainder of this section analyses the existing evidence in terms of what this demonstrates about joint commissioning, but before embarking on this task we try to identify in more detail just what it is that this way of working is supposed to achieve.

Box 10.1: Difficulties in evaluating joint commissioning

- Joint commissioning takes many different forms – how can we be sure we are comparing like with like?
- What do different stakeholders consider to be measures of the success of joint commissioning and what does success look like according to these different perspectives?
- How do the aims of joint commissioning differ from previous arrangements and from other improvement programmes?
- Where do the agendas of partners overlap and form joint work, and what falls outside this collaborative endeavour?
- Which outcome measures are most appropriate to the aims and objectives of joint working?
- What aspects of context have helped/hindered formation and functioning of the joint commissioning arrangement?
- What are the chains of causality/theories underpinning the impact that joint commissioning is intended to have?
- How can unintended consequences be captured?
- Over what timescales do we expect to see outcomes occur?
- How can we be certain that any changes in outcomes are due to joint working and not other influences/policies in the local area?
- Is the local population affected by joint commissioning comparable to that subject to previous service arrangements? Are only the effects on individuals who have received services from the joint services measured?

So what does the evidence say?

A burgeoning literature has emerged that focuses on the processes and practices of joint commissioning, describing how integrated structures have been created and the factors that have helped and hindered the process. Within this evidence there is a debate about whether effective joint commissioning is as a result of the right kind of 'structures' being put in place, or whether it is more to do with the degree of human 'agency' that actors display in overcoming some of the barriers associated with its delivery (Cambridge, 1997, p 29). The literature is largely practice based (rather than empirical studies) and concentrates its efforts on describing the processes used to commission jointly and the types of practices used to overcome any barriers that emerge in implementation.

What is missing from the debate is a discussion about the types of outcomes that different types of joint commissioning processes produce. Instead, studies report 'outputs' such as: the number of newly created integrated services; the number of new housing units providing specialist care (Banks, 2005, p 22); or the strategic efforts being made to generate a shared vision across different policy agendas (Klee, 2009). One integrated organisation recently reported positive progress in achieving outputs such as improved coordination of service delivery and better sharing of information between teams (Valios, 2010), but also highlighted the enormous transaction costs involved in the transfer of staff between agencies. There are, of course, parallels here with the wider literature on health and social care collaboration, where research has often privileged a focus on processes over outcomes (Dickinson, 2008).

In thinking about why there is this focus, we have already argued that the outcomes of joint commissioning have not always been very well defined. As Greig and Poxton (2001b, p 37) demonstrate in relation to care trusts:

> A quick review of the embryonic literature ... reveals that the ... term is used to cover all possible combinations of commissioning [and] providing for any or all client groups or service mixes. Thus a care trust in one place may be concerned solely with commissioning and purchasing older peoples' services, in another be a learning disability provider and in another cover all NHS and social services commissioning as well as social services provision and NHS provision in Mental Health, Learning Disability, older people and community health.

Trying to make a reality of these amorphous outcomes is difficult and often sites retreat to thinking about more tangible issues such as outputs and processes. Often, then, it is claimed that joint commissioning is effective where it has led to the establishment of structures and processes, but not necessarily to better outcomes. Essentially, joint commissioning becomes an end in itself, rather than being a means to specified ends. Of course, there are some shining exceptions to be found, as

Hudson (2010) illustrates, but on the whole, researchers have focused on process over outcome measures (Ramsay and Fulop, 2008). The next subsection stays on the topic of outcomes and investigates in more detail which types of outcomes joint commissioning is aiming to achieve.

What should joint commissioning achieve?

As we have already suggested, joint commissioning has something of a tendency to mean all things to all people. As any basic text in evaluation will tell you, it is incredibly difficult to evaluate something when we do not know what we should be measuring it against. How can we judge it a success, or indeed a failure, if we do not know what we are trying to achieve? This is even more pronounced in terms of joint commissioning as there are likely to be a different array of expectations and values. Furthermore, without a clear idea of what professionals and agencies are attempting to achieve in terms of joint working, then it is hard to attribute change to these activities. As we have already outlined, joint commissioning has often been 'sold' to a wide array of audiences on the basis that it is broadly 'a good thing', but with little more detail about what that 'better thing' actually looks like in practice. This subsection attempts to analyse the policy context and get to grips with what it is that joint commissioning is 'really' attempting to achieve.

Early policy goals to improve joint working between agencies across health and social care were based around the need to reduce the fragmentation or organisational silos that had developed over time, which, it was argued, made it difficult for people with complex care needs to receive the care they required. The joint consultative committees and joint planning groups of the 1970s were statutory bodies largely driven by the need to plan for health and social care services in their local area to overcome issues of organisational fragmentation. However, following the election of the New Labour government in 1997, we witnessed an attempt to shift joint commissioning away from its earlier 'planning' focus through to 'effective partnerships' by 'agreeing a joint strategy through jointly agreed resources' (Greig, 1997, p 27). In the early years of the decade following 2000, joint commissioning took on a more action-oriented feel in contrast to the previous joint planning efforts, but there was still limited advice from central government about how joint commissioning should actually be achieved in practice (Poxton, 1999).

One of the major facilitators of these joint initiatives was introduced in the Health Act 1999. The legislative freedoms known as Section 31 and latterly Section 75 'flexibilities' were introduced as a means of overcoming some of the barriers to effective partnership working. These flexibilities allowed health and social care organisations for the first time (legally at least) to pool budgets, appoint a lead commissioner and set up integrated provider services. Organisations could use one or all of these flexibilities in practice, and a national evaluation found that pooled budgets were the most popular option (Glendinning et al, 2002), albeit that a later study found that pooled budgets only accounted for about 3.4% of total health and social care expenditure (Audit Commission, 2009). One of the main themes of discussions surrounding joint commissioning is this focus on finance, albeit that there is little evidence that joint commissioning is more cost-effective in practice.

The organisational divisions separating health and social care are deep-rooted in longstanding political and administrative arrangements and, arguably, the implications of this division are more than simply structural fragmentation. The UK health and social care system of today is based on the assumption that it is possible to distinguish between people who are 'sick' (and have 'health' needs met free at the point of delivery by the NHS) and people who are merely 'frail' or 'disabled' (who are seen as having 'social care' needs that fall under the remit of means-tested local authority services). Whether an individual has health or social care needs is significant in terms of who pays for services to address these needs and, as a consequence, debates have frequently raged over whether a service user requires 'healthcare' or 'social care'. However, it is argued by commentators such as Glasby (2007) that the distinction between individuals who are 'sick' and those who are 'frail' does not often tend to be meaningful in practice. Particularly for individuals who require long-term care, it is sometimes difficult to be definitive about whether the issue they are trying to get support with is one that is a 'healthcare' or 'social care' need. Consequently, there are a number of accounts of vulnerable individuals and their families who have attempted to access services or support from the public sector and found that care is subject to debates over who should pay, is uncoordinated, is of poor quality or, in some cases, is non-existent (see, for example, Glasby and Littlechild, 2004; Henwood, 2006).

By pooling budgets across health and social care, then, it is anticipated that these types of debates should be consigned to the past. There will no longer be incentives for health and social care agencies to 'cost-shunt' to their partner and therefore make it difficult for service users to access care. It is also argued that single agency models of commissioning provide little incentive for social care or primary and community care services to invest in services that they see few returns on. For example, as part of a joined-up approach to commissioning, partners might agree to invest in preventative low-level services that aim to save money on expensive acute medical services in the future. Whereas in the past, social care might traditionally commission and fund these activities, PCTs might agree to invest in these services as a way to prevent admissions to acute or institutional care settings. Similarly, local authorities might invest in PCT intermediate care services as a means of reintroducing individuals to the community after a hospital stay and preventing a residential care admission. Although there is some evidence emerging around preventative services, this is limited in practice – particularly in terms of joint commissioning.

The idea of joint commissioning having an impact on cost-effectiveness might also happen in another sense beyond that of prevention. By aligning needs assessments, partners might reduce duplication in terms of overlap of services that are provided by both health and social care agencies. Furthermore, streamlining assessment processes might also deliver cost-effectiveness. The virtue of simply having pooled budgets might provide what Hastings (1996) refers to as 'resource synergy', essentially the idea that larger budgets are more cost-effective as they allow more power and 'bang for the buck'. Again, though, the degree to which this has been achieved in practice is limited.

So far we have made the argument that an interest in joint commissioning has been driven by: the structural fragmentation that has resulted in divisions between agencies involved in the design and delivery of health and social care; an attempt to promote cost-effectiveness; and as a means of promoting prevention. However, there is another recent agenda that has gained much interest in health and social care: personalisation (see also Chapter Eleven, this volume). Recently, much attention has been given to the relationship between service users and health and social care agencies as reforms have sought to 'place people at the centre of commissioning' through involving patients in the design and delivery of health and social care services (DH, 2007a). These attempts to shift power away from professionals towards service users imply a new form of 'joining up services' – and one that is driven by service users. As Dickinson and Glasby (2008) argue, joint commissioning becomes imperative under this situation in order that health and social care agencies might be able to support the type of market stimulating and managing activities that are necessary and also be able to deal with the issue of risk effectively.

In addition to viewing service users as potential additional 'partners' in joint commissioning, policy has also sought to extend beyond health and social care to other stakeholders. One of the main critiques that was made of early attempts at joint commissioning was that partners wider than health and social care were often not involved in these processes (Cambridge, 1997). Hence, when the Office for Public Management (2008, p 28) talks about operational commissioning in the context of children's services, it specifies a much broader focus on 'localities or groups of children with similar needs' involving schools, groups of schools, GPs and partnerships delivering services for children such as Child and Adolescent Mental Health Services (CAMHS) or Youth Offending Teams. In recent years there has also been an increased interest in the notion of strategic commissioning, 'Total Place' and 'place shaping'. This agenda speaks to the idea that services should go beyond simply overseeing a collection of public services that are delivered in an area and should become more actively involved in actually influencing and supporting that area (Lyons, 2004). As such, some commentators have argued that relationships between health and social care need to go 'beyond joint commissioning' (Glasby et al, 2010) and not just deliver services to a public in a silo fashion, but do so in a more active way that contributes to the very fabric of a local area.

As we have sought to demonstrate in this section, there are many different types of definition of joint commissioning and also an array of different policy drivers that influence why partners may feel that they should engage in these activities (summarised in Table 10.2). Inevitably, it is difficult to be clear about a policy agenda where there are so many different potential meanings and implications.

Table 10.2: The many drivers of joint commissioning

Driver	Explanation
Organisational fragmentation	Due to the structural fragmentation that is experienced between health and social care it is crucial that health and social care agencies work together in order to overcome the difficulties that service users encounter in navigating services
Cost-effectiveness	Joint commissioning should lead to a reduction of duplication between health and social care agencies and a streamlining of assessment processes. Joint budgets should also lead to 'resource synergy'
Prevention	Joint commissioning should facilitate preventative services by engaging a range of different statutory and non-statutory agencies in activities that provide low-level support, which should reduce the need for expensive acute or institutional care
Personalisation	If service users are to be able to direct their support in a truly personalised way then joint commissioning is needed to stimulate/manage markets and provide the support that these 'micro-commissioners' need
Place shaping	Health and social care services should play a role with other partners in not just passively delivering services, but also actively shaping the nature of that geographical locality

In a number of ways, these observations illustrate the types of debates that go on in relation to the broader notion of health and social care collaboration. This is important, as definitions of joint commissioning are often not set out explicitly, and this notion is conflated with the issue of health and social collaboration in its broadest sense. Against this background, some responsibility for defining key concepts, approaches and desired outcomes must lie with local agencies when exploring what arrangements to develop and the types of impacts they are trying to achieve. Without this sort of knowledge it becomes difficult to be definitive about the outcomes of joint commissioning, and there is a risk that it becomes an end in itself (rather than a means to an end).

Conclusions

'Joint commissioning' has remained an important concept in policy over time. In order to provide more effective, joined-up and preventative services that support well-being, it is argued that joint commissioning is crucial. Yet, it is not clear either what is meant by joint commissioning or what it is supposed to deliver in practice. Beyond broad notions that joint commissioning should lead to better outcomes, there is limited evidence of this in the literature. Although there is some evidence relating to the types of practices and processes that are associated with joint commissioning, there is rather less in the way of outcomes. In a number of ways there are parallels between the key points of debate in the joint commissioning literature and the wider literature on joint working (with which discussions of joint commissioning are often conflated). The implications of this are that local organisations should be clear about what it is they are trying to achieve when engaging in joint commissioning, and there needs to be more research that looks at outcomes and which can give us a better insight into what the impacts of joint commissioning may actually be.

Further reading

This is a topic where much of the literature is descriptive and where many of the main texts lack an underlying evidence base. However, helpful resources include:

- Department of Health (1995) *Practical guidance on joint commissioning for project leaders*, London: Department of Health – roots the origins of joint commissioning in better partnership working between health and social care agencies.
- Department of Health (2007) *Commissioning framework for health and well-being*, London, Department of Health – describes the more recent policy shift that has occurred away from partnerships between health and social care agencies towards those with a wider health and well-being agenda. It also introduces strategic needs assessment as a policy tool.
- Dickinson, H. (2008) *Evaluating outcomes in health and social care*, Bristol: The Policy Press – provides background discussion of some of the practical difficulties associated with evaluating partnerships, and offers a useful basis for understanding the complexities that arise when trying to assess the impact of joint commissioning on service user and carer outcomes.
- Edwards, M. and Miller, C. (2003) *Integrating health and social care and making it work*, London: Office for Public Management (Chapter 1: The policy context) – explains the historical context of policy tools to promote joint commissioning such as the Health Act 1999 flexibilities.
- Rummery, K. and Glendinning, C. (2000) *Primary care and social services: developing new partnerships for older people*, Oxford: Radcliffe Medical Press (Chapter 1: Partnerships between primary care and social care) – provides a useful backdrop to some of the historical context to joint commissioning, describing how the health/social care divide has emerged and its subsequent impact on service users, carers and their families.

Useful websites

- NHS Evidence – provides a comprehensive range of online web resources linked to joint commissioning and commissioning in health and social care settings: www.library.nhs.uk/healthmanagement/viewresource.aspx?resid=262514
- Integrated Care Network – provides online resources to frontline staff working in health and social care seeking to improve outcomes for service users: www. dhcarenetworks.org.uk/Integration/icn/aboutICN/ (content now archived)
- Strategic Commissioning Development Unit (SCDU) – a health-based resource providing 'commissioning packs' for frontline commissioners in a range of clinical areas: www.dh.gov.uk/en/Publicationsandstatistics/Publications/PublicationsPolicyAndGuidance/Browsable/DH_117500

Reflective exercises

1. Whichever area of health and social care you work in or are studying, read a recent policy document on joint working/joint commissioning. Using Table 10.2, what are the key drivers towards joint commissioning and what do policy makers or local leaders seem to be hoping that joint commissioning will achieve?
2. Where you have read about, visited or worked in a service that is jointly commissioned, how 'joint' does it feel in practice and what is the service achieving that a service commissioned by a single agency might not have been able to deliver?
3. Talk to local service users and/or health and social care practitioners. What do they understand by the term 'joint commissioning' and what do they want jointly commissioned services to achieve on their behalf?
4. As public finances have become much more restricted following the economic problems of 2009/10, what impact will this have on joint commissioning?

References

Allen, B.A., Wade, E. and Dickinson, H. (2009) 'Bridging the divide – commercial procurement and supply chain management: are there lessons for health care commissioning in England?', *Journal of Public Procurement*, vol 9, pp 505-34.

Audit Commission (2009) *Means to an end: joint financing across health and social care*, London: Audit Commission.

Banks, P. (2002) *Partnerships under pressure: a commentary on progress in partnership-working between the NHS and local government*, London: King's Fund.

Banks, P. (2005) 'New hurdles for integrated commissioning', *Journal of Integrated Care*, vol 13, pp 21-6.

Beveridge, W. (1942) *Social insurance and allied services*, Cmnd 6404, London: HMSO.

Cambridge, D. (1997) 'Commentary: joint commissioning: searching for stability in an unstable world', *Tizard Learning Disability Review*, vol 2, pp 26-30.

DH (Department of Health) (1989) *Working for patients*, London: HMSO.

DH (1995) *An introduction to joint commissioning*, London: DH.

DH (1998) *Partnership in action: new opportunities for joint working between health and social services*, London: HMSO.

DH (2007a) *Commissioning framework for health and wellbeing*, London: DH.

DH (2007b) *Guidance on Joint strategic needs assessment*, London: DH.

DH (2010) *Equity and excellence: liberating the NHS*, London: TSO.

Dickinson, H. (2008) *Evaluating outcomes in health and social care*, Bristol: The Policy Press.

Dickinson, H. and Glasby, J. (2008) 'Not throwing out the partnership agenda with the personalisation bathwater', *Journal of Integrated Care*, vol 16, pp 3-8.

Dowling, B., Powell, M. and Glendinning, C. (2004) 'Conceptualising successful partnerships', *Health and Social Care in the Community*, vol 12, pp 309-17.

Glasby, J. (2007) *Understanding health and social care*, Bristol: The Policy Press.

Glasby, J. and Dickinson, H. (2008) *Partnership working in health and social care*, Bristol: The Policy Press.

Glasby, J. and Littlechild, R. (2004) *The health and social care divide*, Bristol: The Policy Press.

Glasby, J., Dickinson, H. and Smith, J. (2010) 'Creating "NHS Local": the relationship between English local government and the National Health Service', *Social Policy and Administration*, vol 44, pp 244-64.

Glendinning, C., Rummery, K. and Clarke, R. (1998) 'From collaboration to commissioning: developing relationships between primary health and social services', *British Medical Journal*, vol 323, pp 122-25.

Glendinning, C., Hudson, B., Hardy, B. and Young, R. (2002) *National evaluation of notifications for the use of the Section 31 partnership flexibilities in the Health Act 1999: final project report*, Leeds and Manchester: Nuffield Institute for Health/National Primary Care Research and Development Centre.

Greig, R. (1997) 'Joint commissioning: searching for stability in an unstable world', *Tizard Learning Disability Review*, vol 2, pp 19-25.

Greig, R. and Poxton, R. (2001a) 'Nice process – But did joint commissioning change anyone's life?', *Managing Community Care*, vol 9, no 2, pp 16-32.

Greig, R. and Poxton, R. (2001b) 'From joint commissioning to partnership working – will the new policy framework make a difference?', *Managing Community Care*, vol 9, pp 32-8.

Hastings, A. (1996) 'Unravelling the process of 'partnership' in urban regeneration policy', *Urban Studies*, vol 33, pp 253-68.

Henwood, M. (2006) 'The treatment gap', *Society Guardian*, 31 May, p 6.

Hudson, B. (1999) 'Joint commissioning across the primary health care – social care boundary: can it work?', *Health and Social Care in the Community*, vol 7, no 5, pp 358-66.

Hudson, B. (2010) 'Integrated commissioning: new context, new dilemmas, new solutions?', *Journal of Integrated Care*, vol 18, pp 11-19.

Hudson, B. and Willis, J. (1995) *Analysis of joint commissioning developments in the Northern region*, Leeds: Nuffield Institute for Health.

Kerslake, A. (2007) *An approach to outcome-based commissioning and contracting*, London: CSIP.

Klee, D. (2009) 'Reconciling Putting People First and world class commissioning: a case study', *Journal of Integrated Care*, vol 17, 27-34.

Lyons, M. (2004) *Shaping the pattern of government service: independent review of public sector relocation*, London: HM Treasury.

Office for Public Management (2008) *Literature review: multi-level commissioning*, London: OPM.

Poxton, R. (1999) *Working across boundaries*, London: King's Fund.

Ramsay, A. and Fulop, N. (2008) *The evidence base for integrated care*, London: Department of Health.

Rummery, K. and Glendinning, C. (2000) *Primary care and social services: developing new partnerships for older people*, Oxford: Radcliffe Medical Press.

Smith, J., Mays, N., Dixon, J., Goodwin, N., Lewis, R., McClelland, S., McLeod, H. and Wyke, S. (2004) *A review of the effectiveness of primary care-led commissioning and its place in the NHS*, London: The Health Foundation.

Timmins, N. (2001) *The five giants: a biography of the welfare state*, London: HarperCollins.

Valios, N. (2010) 'The pros and cons of care trusts for adult care', *Community Care*, 1 March, www.communitycare.co.uk/Articles/2010/03/04/113954/the-pros-and-cons-of-care-trusts-for-adult-care.htm

Walshe, K., Smith, J., Dixon, J., Edwards, N., Hunter, D. J., Mays, N., Normand, C. and Robinson, R. (2004) 'Primary care trusts – premature reorganisation, with mergers, may be harmful', *British Medical Journal*, vol 329, pp 871-72.

ELEVEN

Commissioning in an era of personalisation

Catherine Needham and Simon Duffy

Summary

This chapter explores:
- the emergence and spread of personalisation;
- issues for commissioners;
- experiences from frontline practice;
- the future of personalised commissioning.

Personalisation constitutes a new approach to the delivery of public services, which will create profound challenges for all aspects of their provision, including commissioning. Although definitions of personalisation vary, there is a general agreement that it involves 'a shift from access to the uniform to access to the individualised' (Cutler et al, 2007, p 850). To achieve this requires 'thinking about public services ... in an entirely different way – starting with the person rather than the service' (Carr, 2010, p 67). Personalised approaches are furthest developed in social care, but they are spreading rapidly into other services, including health. The change of government in Westminster has seen no let-up in the pace of implementation, as the Liberal-Conservative coalition has expressed itself to be as keen on personalised approaches as its New Labour predecessors (HM Government, 2010). The broad coalition of support behind personalisation makes Mansell and Beadle-Brown's (2005, p 21) observation seem ever more apt: 'there is now no serious alternative to the principle that services should be tailored to individual needs, circumstances and wants'.

This chapter focuses on the implications of personalisation for commissioning in health and social care. In particular, it explores the impact of individualised forms of budget control (particularly personal budgets in social care) on the commissioning process. As service users increasingly commission their own services, this creates new challenges for local authorities as their roles shift from the negotiation of block and spot contracts to the stimulating and shaping of local markets. With personalised budgets being piloted in children's services and in healthcare, a number of commentators are beginning to wonder whether such new commissioning models will spread from adult social care to other areas of the welfare state, with personalisation becoming a new 'organising logic' for the early 21st century, as influential as privatisation was in previous eras (Leadbeater, 2004, pp 18-19).

The chapter begins by exploring the emergence of personalisation in social care, looking at the introduction of direct payments in the mid–1990s and the development of individual and personal budgets after 2003. It discusses the spread of personalisation into other sectors, identifying its potential to reshape commissioning in health, housing, education, employment services and criminal justice. The chapter then considers the issues that personalised approaches to commissioning are likely to generate, before looking at some specific examples of implementation experiences in the social care sector. It concludes by considering the future challenges that personalisation will pose for commissioners.

From direct payments to Putting People First

The principle that disabled people could commission their own services rather than relying on professionally determined allocations, emerged from a number of campaigns from the early 1980s. Challenging the norm of institutional living, insights from the independent living movement and the social model of disability provided an entirely different paradigm in which people were recognised to be 'experts on their own lives' (Poll, 2007, p 53). Control over resources came to be a key demand of disability campaigners, on the assumption that people knew better than professionals how to allocate funds most effectively. Early experimentation with cash allocations to disabled people or third parties by local authorities (of dubious legality) eventually contributed to the case for change, with the Major government accepting that care legislation should be changed to make direct payments lawful (Leece and Bornat, 2006). The passage of the Community Care (Direct Payments) Act 1996 gave local authorities the power to make direct payments. This became a duty in England and Wales in 2001 and in Scotland in 2003. The payments were initially available for younger disabled people (aged 18–65), and later extended to include older people, disabled children, people lacking mental capacity and carers.

Take-up of direct payments was relatively limited, however, constituting a small minority of potential users (Leece and Bornat, 2006). From 2003, the social innovation network In Control worked with local authorities to develop self-directed approaches, including individual budgets, which integrated funding from a wider range of sources than direct payments and could be spent more creatively (Poll et al, 2006). Interest in the individual budget approach from a number of government departments led the Department of Health to pilot individual budgets in 13 councils from 2005. Evaluation of the pilots found that the initiative was generally welcomed by participants, who reported feeling that they had more control over their daily lives (Glendinning et al, 2008). However, attempts to integrate multiple budget streams were found to be problematic, as a result of which mainstream implementation has focused on developing personal budgets for social care.

The Putting People First concordat was signed in 2007 between central government, local government and the social care sector, marking a new level of commitment to personalising social care. The concordat widened the personalisation agenda, emphasising that it should not just be seen as personal budgets or direct payments (HM Government, 2007). Personalisation was to be about choice and control for the individual, with a number of strands, including early intervention and prevention (linked to reablement), social capital and improved access to universal services. A three-year transforming social care grant of £520 million was allocated to local authorities from 2008, to assist in the move to personalised care. Putting People First called for all eligible users to have access to a personal budget, although a later national government performance measure (National Indicator 130) set a transitional target for 30% to be on personal budgets by April 2011. The government has since affirmed that it expects all eligible users to have access to a personal budget by 2012. The budget can be held in part or whole by the user (or a nominated representative) as a direct payment, or continue to be managed by the local authority. Most local authorities are currently setting up a resource allocation system (RAS) to calculate the amount of money a service user can receive in a personal budget, with many opting for a RAS developed by In Control.

Personalisation beyond social care

The perceived success of personalisation in adult social care – with early results suggesting improved outcomes for budget holders at no increased cost (Tyson et al, 2010) – has led to widespread interest in the scope for similar approaches to be used in other sectors of the welfare state. In children's social care, for example, In Control has worked with 22 children's services to explore the potential for personal budgets and the wider personalisation agenda for children, young people and families, through the Taking Control programme (Crosby, 2010). The-then Department for Education and Skills launched pilots to provide individual budgets for disabled children and their families through the Aiming High programme (DfES, 2007). At a regional level, Yorkshire and Humber have supported work improving the experiences of young people at the point of transition to adult services, including working with special schools to support person-centred planning (Cowen, 2010). For children with additional needs, which may include having a physical or learning disability, speaking English as a second language or being at risk of abuse or neglect, there have been pilots of a budget-holding lead professional (BHLP) model. This approach releases resources to the front line without making users themselves directly responsible for budget management. Staff nominated as a BHLP help to coordinate a wide range of services and to work creatively with families and other staff to access resources (OPM, 2008).

Moves to make the National Health Service (NHS) more personalised, through the expansion of choice, improved access and the recognition of the scope for people with long-term conditions to act as 'expert patients', have been under way for several years. Personal health budgets, along the lines of personal budgets for social care, had been rejected in a 2006 White Paper (DH, 2006) for compromising the free at the point of use principles of NHS funding. However the Darzi reviews of the NHS, published in 2007 and 2008, revived the idea of individual budgets, reflecting their perceived success in social care (Darzi 2007, 2008). The budgets are currently being piloted in a range of services, including mental health, maternity, end-of life care and substance abuse (DH, 2009a). Patients can opt to manage the money themselves, following new legislation on direct payments in health. Alternatively, they can work with health professionals or a third party to identify how to allocate a notional or managed budget. There has been a high level of interest, with 75 primary care trusts (PCTs) expressing interest in developing a pilot, for a range of services. Running alongside the personal health budget pilots is an In Control initiative – 'Staying in Control' – which is examining how personalisation models developed within social care can best be amended and tested within the NHS (see www.in-control.org.uk/health).

Personalisation is less developed in other public services, although there is widespread interest in how it might be incorporated. This includes discussion of the scope for supported housing to be more personalised, as part of the commitment to personalisation within social care. Under the government's Think Family initiative, oriented towards families at risk, housing is one element that can be included in an individual budget (Taylor Knox, 2009, p 17). Local authorities can also draw on Supporting People funds, which provide housing support for vulnerable people, to offer personalised support (Audit Commission, 2009). The government has noted the possibility of using personal budgets to provide options for 'some marginalized groups including the small numbers of people who have slept rough for many years and have, up to now, been unwilling to accept the help on offer' (DH Care Networks, 2009). There is also some interest in how the third sector can be more involved in offering tailored approaches to offender management and reducing reoffending (ACEVO, 2009; Concilium, 2009).

Within employment services, the Department for Work and Pensions has developed a programme of 'personalised conditionality', stating its intention to 'provide support that is tailored to each person's needs and to give everyone the opportunity to develop skills so they can find, and get on in, work' (DWP, 2008, p 11). For disabled jobseekers there has been a commitment to provide greater control over the money spent on their behalf – linking up to the broader personalisation agenda in social care. Legislation in 2009 introduced Right to Control Trailblazer pilots, which will integrate resources from a range of funds, including Work Choice and Access to Work, aimed at facilitating entry to the workforce for disabled people (DWP, 2008).

Personalised learning within schools has been on the agenda for several years (Miliband, 2004), although there may be tensions with the national curriculum and testing programme (Campbell et al, 2007). Some new academies have experimented with more creative approaches to school buildings and timetabling

(SSAT, 2010). The new government's intention to make individual pupil funding more transparent, for example, in relation to the pupil premium for disadvantaged children, may signal a shift in emphasis that makes devolved forms of funding possible (Gove, 2010).

Given the scope for personalisation to transform many sectors of the welfare state, Glasby et al (2010) have suggested that it may constitute an alternative model to the Beveridgian welfare settlement. As more resources are controlled directly by citizens, or by those working closely with them, it may be possible to rethink the tax and benefit system such that contributions and entitlements of citizens could be simplified (Duffy, 2010). A 'Conditional Resource Entitlement', in which government targets resources towards eligible individuals with specific conditions attached, could be used in a wider range of sectors (Duffy et al, 2010).

Although personalisation is at an early stage of development in many of these sectors, it is evident that the sorts of approaches it encompasses – involving more tailoring to individual users, a more diverse range of non-state providers and the disaggregation of budgets to the individual level – are likely to create a number of challenges for traditional commissioning models. The next section sets out what some of these challenges are likely to be, before going on to offer some reflections from the practice context within social care.

Issues for commissioners

Local authority commissioning on a large scale is relatively new, emerging from the community care reforms of the early 1990s. However, the personalised commissioning model requires another rethinking of the local authority role. In the new model, commissioning will not be limited to people 'with commissioning in their job title' (DH, 2008), but will be done by service users and staff on behalf of users, drawing on a wider than ever range of providers. Rather than commissioning lying at the heart of 'what the public sector does', as Glasby puts it in the Introduction to this book, it will be increasingly what citizens do for themselves. Reflecting on this, a local authority social care manager commented, 'We need to stop using the language of commissioning. People won't "commission" things – they will buy them' (Needham, 2010, p 34).

To understand this new context it is helpful to draw on the nested view of commissioning developed by the Department of Health, in which individual purchasing by service users links to operational commissioning (in which local authority or PCT commissioners shape local markets and support service users), and above that to strategic commissioning at area and regional levels (DH, 2008).

If existing managers and commissioners are to realise the vision of personalisation, it will require being responsive to the diverse ways in which users want services to be personalised, with some choosing to manage a budget and others wanting traditional services to be delivered in a more flexible way. Commissioners are expected to be responsive to carers, self-funders and future users, as well as existing users (HM Government, 2007). This requires dealing with the conflicting needs that these groups will sometimes have, identifying ways of recognising and responding to conflicting priorities (for example balancing user preferences for flexible, community-based services, with carer needs for regular and predictable short breaks). They are also expected to be alert to opportunities for preventative funding and reablement in order to improve outcomes and cut costs.

Commissioners must oversee the creation of a new infrastructure of support planners (or brokers) if individual purchasing is to be a reality. There are various models available for this, including local authority-based support planners, independent brokers, advocates from user-led organisations or other third sector organisations, or informal support from peers and family (Duffy and Fulton, 2009). All of these approaches will necessitate different funding models, and imply a different power balance between stakeholders. There appears to be little support for a new profession of independent broker (Dowson and Greig, 2009; Duffy and Fulton, 2009), with most local authorities proving support in-house or leaving it to third sector organisations or peer support networks. In some areas, local authority in-house support planning is being funded through top-slicing personal budgets. Often it is existing care managers who do both the assessments and the support planning, although the Department of Health has recommended that the roles be kept separate. In other areas, third sector organisations such as Centres for Independent Living are playing a key role in providing support. Some third sector organisations currently fund their own advice and advocacy services and are waiting for clarification about how these services will be funded in the more uncertain financial climate of individual purchasing. There are also concerns over conflicts of interest where organisations provide both brokerage and services, and some third sector organisations are setting up a separate social enterprise arm to minimise the conflict.

As more and more service users commission their own services, local authority commissioners will be expected to draw together (and share with providers) intelligence about the state of the local market and demographic data about current and future demand for services. A key role at this operational level will be working with providers on business development skills, market responsiveness and financial planning. This involves responding to a wide range of providers with very diverse needs – from large-scale private and third sector providers, used to relying on block contracts, to micro-providers and user-led organisations that may offer very different services and have very different financial and organisational needs to the larger providers. Providers will need support in making the transition from 'wholesale to retail' provision, and in the new roles they are required to play in relation to care management, human resources management and support planning. Providers may be offered outcome-focused contracts in place of task- and time-based contracts, designed to assure quality and supply through the pre-selection or validation of providers (DH, 2009b). Decisions need to be made about local accreditation practices for personal assistants and providers; many local authorities are still consulting locally on whether to create a register of personal assistants. There is a trade-off to be made here between maintaining a skilled and trained base of personal assistants and the freedom that budget holders may want to make their own choices about who to employ.

Local authorities and external providers will need to become more effective in pricing services, ensuring that costs are covered at a level that reflects what people are willing to pay. For some providers already providing services to self-funders or to the wider community, individual pricing models will be well developed. However, there may be many services, provided in-house by local authorities or by external providers, which have previously been bundled together and/or purchased on a block contract basis, which will need to be disaggregated. New internal systems will be required to link pricing to unit costs.

A further challenge for commissioners will be to decommission some existing services in order to release resources for personal budgets. In some areas, day centres are already closing on the basis that they cannot be funded if some users withdraw their funding. Many people will not regret their passing, seeing them as offering a very limited vision of how disabled people might want to spend their time. However, there are concerns about what happens to people who continue to want day centre provision that is no longer available, and about the individualisation of users who lack collective spaces to come together. A review of the Department of Health's Valuing People Now strategy for people with learning disabilities highlighted the continuing need for 'a local base from which people can access different activities' (Mansell, 2010, p 29). For local politicians there are also difficult political battles about closing high-profile centres of long standing.

More broadly, commissioners must work to ensure that personalisation is a model for a fuller citizenship rather than a tool for individualisation and atomisation. A number of authors have noted the scope for personalisation to enrich rather than weaken connections to the community, as people have scope to access universal services rather than segregated provision (Keohane, 2009; Duffy, 2010). In part, this reflects a broader concern within the personalisation debate about the role that social capital should play alongside funded state support. A key element of personalisation within social care has been around helping people to develop networks of support that are based on friendship and reciprocity rather than contract. A HACT (formerly the Housing Associations' Charitable Trust) project on service user purchasing consortia for people with individual budgets and/or direct payments points to the ways in which commissioners can support more integrated approaches (see http://hact.org.uk/up2us).

As well as supporting individual commissioning, and ensuring effective operational interventions, there is a challenge for local authorities and related bodies to ensure effective strategic commissioning for their localities. The central imperative at the strategic level appears to be integrated commissioning between health and social care, perhaps as part of combined individual budgets spanning health and care services (Allen et al, 2009; HM Government, 2010). The importance of joint working between local agencies has been emphasised by a number of government initiatives, including Local Strategic Partnerships, Local Area Agreements, the former Comprehensive Area Assessment and Total

Place. There are clear linkages between place-based budgeting approaches and the personalisation agenda. As Duffy (2010, p 12) puts it, 'Personalisation offers an ideal set of technologies to enable a Total Place strategy to work – because it offers a flexible framework for putting resources in the hands of citizens, families and communities. It also enables fresh conversations between citizens and the state about what really needs to be achieved.'

Personalisation requires commissioners, providers and users to encounter new forms of risk, and at a strategic level there is a need to identify and manage this process. For providers, there will be organisational and financial risks posed by the new retail model, in which the security of local authority block contracts will disappear. Private and third sector providers need to identify ways to manage this new risk profile, and to work with local authorities to minimise the risk of market failure (perhaps through accessing preferred provider status). Local authorities and other commissioning bodies need to manage the risks of market failure. Some local authorities are anticipating and putting in place contingency funding for market failure – although this may be a big drain on resources. Commissioning organisations will also need to clarify how far they can (or should) divest themselves of legal liability for the spending choices of people with personal budgets, for example if there are legal disputes between direct payment holders and personal assistants, or if people choose to purchase inappropriate support services (ADASS, 2009).

The broader relationship between safeguarding and personalisation is not yet clear. There are risks relating to the potential for abuse of budget holders, informal carers or employees. This also includes the potential for misuse of public monies, as service users opt for non-traditional spending. Getting the regulation right for personalisation – avoiding excessive audit and regulation mechanisms while providing appropriate protections – will be a difficult balance. Social workers may feel more exposed as they sign off support plans over which they have less control than traditional care plans, fearing that they will retain responsibility if things go wrong. There will need to be a certain amount of courage from managers and politicians when the media gets hold of a story about abuse of a budget. As just one example, adverse coverage of personal budgets allegedly being spent on 'prostitutes for the disabled' indicates growing media attention on how budgets are being used and monitored (Donnelly et al, 2010).

Experiences from frontline practice

Interviews with politicians, civil servants, local authority managers, frontline staff, service users and carers, trades union representatives, academics, consultants and staff from private and third sector providers, have highlighted some of the commissioning challenges currently being experienced in the social care sector (Needham, 2010). These include:

Lack of information

There are concerns that local commissioners lack the knowledge that is needed to make markets work. One national policy officer in a voluntary organisation felt that local authorities do not have basic market knowledge: "You can only stimulate the market if you know what your provider market is, the vast majority of local authorities don't actually know the massive amounts of activity that are going on in their local authority areas anyway." Commissioners too are concerned that they do not have the right skills for market shaping: "A sophisticated approach is required to manage a market, you need analysis and modelling skills. We don't have that" (local authority social care manager). Another manager said "It is quite difficult to stimulate a market in a context of personalisation because there is less security."

The costing and pricing of services is one issue where information is lacking. As one third sector provider put it, "At the moment we can't see the cost of the in-house day centres, so we've got nothing to compare with." Uncertainty about costing is often internal as well as external, with local authority staff themselves not having access to disaggregated costings for their services (OPM, 2008, p 40). Support planners, who are supposed to advise budget holders on their spending choices, do not always have a clear sense of what may and may not be funded using a personal budget. One support planner expressed her frustration with her local authority employer: "You ask questions but no one knows the answer." According to another, "We need more support on knowing what we should be funding and what not, what people should have a responsibility for paying for themselves." A manager from a user-led organisation for disabled people commented "The support planners don't know how to cost things, they don't understand that personal assistants have overheads, like holiday and sick pay."

Undeveloped services

Even if local authority commissioners get better at mapping local markets, there may well be inadequate provision available in the local setting. As one social care manager put it, "Our sense at the moment is that the market is very dysfunctional. There are few incentives for providers to be innovative. I don't know of any authority that can genuinely say otherwise." According to another, "People say to us it's all very well to have direct payments but there's bugger all to buy" (director of adult social care, local authority). Although personalisation envisages that dynamic new markets will emerge in response to budget holder demands, there are dangers that local markets will contract rather than grow as providers lose the security of block contracts. Another interviewee reflected on the issues: "It's going to take a lot of fleetness of foot and commitment from commissioners, both local authority and health, to make sure you don't idiotically and unintentionally sweep away some really good services" (civil servant, mental health). Some providers may choose to exit the market altogether. A civil servant working on personalisation and housing warned "Larger providers have made announcements that they are not going for new housing. They are saying that personalisation challenges their care and support packages – pensions, employment rights etc."

Part of the challenge for local authority commissioners will be in striking a balance between helping valued local providers to manage the transition and overseeing the closure of services that no longer meet local need. Interviewees reported that progress on the decommissioning agenda was slow. A local authority chief executive reflected on the pace of change: "Why is the agenda going so slow? It's redundancy costs, it's fear, organisational inertia, not wanting to close down the day centre, or other service. We need to actively manage decommissioning at the same time as giving out budgets." A local authority social care manager said "Personalisation doesn't yet link to decommissioning of services because there isn't yet anything to replace it. We would have thought we'd have a major closure programme for day centres but we aren't because we haven't got a viable alternative offer."

It is anticipated that people with personal budgets might not want to give up day services altogether, but rather to opt in on a more ad hoc basis, attending on particular days or for particular events (Duffy, 2010). More transparent, individualised pricing would allow people to compare the cost of a day centre session with other spending choices, and to decide how much of their weekly budget they wanted to commit to it. However, some interviewees were concerned about how accommodation-based services could be sustained on this basis, given the building and staffing costs of keeping a centre open. There were fears that a few service users choosing to withdraw their funding could lead to the closure of a service that was popular with other users. As one third sector provider put it, "If people want to go to activities like a day centre occasionally, they won't be there. You can't run a day centre on that basis." One director of adult social care was more upbeat about the changes: "We need to demolish the old buildings, cash in their value, and build state-of-the-art facilities for those people who really need them."

In the meantime, a number of local authorities are running two systems in parallel: flexible services for people with personal budgets and traditional day services for people on conventional funding streams. There are clear challenges in operating dual systems at a time of severe budgetary constraint. The Department of Health expects dual operating to be phased out as personal budget holders become a majority of users (DH, 2009b). The national programme manager for Putting People First explained that the target of 30% of eligible people on personal budgets by 2011 is expressly designed to move away from this: "When you have got three or four people on direct payments you can run two systems. We want to ensure self-directed support is the main system" (speaking at an In Control event, 16 March 2010). However, the transitional phase may be a long one. As one interviewee noted, "In local authorities that have relied on block contracts it may take 10 to 15 years to implement – although they've only got a three-year transformation grant."

Lack of integration

One of the key challenges for existing commissioners is to look at the needs of the whole person, rather than just their care or health needs. According to one policy consultant: 'Personalisation, unlike consumerism, focuses on life, not on services.... There will be lots of services that I need – health, education, employment – which are not paid for by a personal budget, but which need to be personalised.' This requires local authorities to develop system-wide approaches to personalisation rather than seeing it as a social care policy. However, one local authority chief executive reported that personalisation remained "ghettoised" in social care. Another interviewee observed "Lots of local authorities have used the transforming social care grant to set up a personalisation team, and then the rest of the local authority and the rest of the adult social care department leave it to that team to bring about personalisation." Voluntary sector interviewees similarly complained that too much of the transforming social care grant has been absorbed by the local authority rather than used to support providers making the transition to personalised services, a concern echoed in a recent report from private sector care providers (ECCA, 2010).

Lack of trust

Local authorities are expected to work closely with providers to manage the transition to personalised commissioning. However, relationships have traditionally been adversarial and many continue to be problematic. As one local authority manager put it: "[Providers] want us to tell them what to do. It's a parent–child relationship, we've been their biggest purchaser. The bulk of providers don't even come to our events." A director of adult social care noted "We're not awash with entrepreneurial spirit here, really." The provider perspective is rather different: "There's local authorities that I'm aware of that are going out doing these pilot activities and are just not talking to the [third] sector.... They come to the provider market and say you've got to do it, it's adapt or die, and that doesn't really work" (national policy officer, voluntary organisation).

Lack of trust is not only an issue affecting local authority–provider relations. There are also indications that service users do not hold local authority managers and care staff in high esteem, and that the feeling may be mutual. One service user noted: "There's lots of suspicion of the local authority.... Because it's the council, people assume there is an agenda behind it." For their part, social care managers found the contribution of service users problematic. As one social care manager put it, "The problem with engagement is that service users just become a lobby group for existing services. They don't see that they have a role in the solution." According to one local authority social care manager, 'Engagement with service users means they come and complain – they are a feisty group. If you go from a high-cost package to a medium-cost package that may be better linked to outcomes for that person, they just see it as a cut." A local authority chief executive made a similar point: "Service users capture the value of the service for themselves and want more of it. We need leading-edge users saying we will do this differently."

Lack of money

Social care has long been afflicted with a lack of investment, but the current financial context imposes even more stringent limitations than in the past. As one local authority social care manager noted, "The circumstances are very different than when we had the national pilot here for personalisation. That was very laissez-faire, very flexible. It had a lot of money thrown at it. Now for older people, personalisation is costing more and we need to look at that." To date, the relationship between personalisation and cuts remains unclear. There is some cynicism that personalisation is being used as a label to legitimise service changes that are more about cutting budgets than about enhancing choice and control. As one policy consultant put it, "Local authorities that are cutting everything, that have massive budget issues, use personalisation and individual budgets to justify anything that they want to do."

Short-term pressures for savings may choke those elements of personalisation that are likely to deliver longer-term savings, such as prevention, early intervention and reablement. One local authority manager explained the challenge: "Personalisation has got to save us money, we've got no choice.... We know we can achieve dramatic savings on individual people. Personalised services will be cheaper in some circumstances, particularly for learning disability and physical disabilities. There's not so much savings to be made on older people because we're stingy to start with." Another was more positive: "Personalisation meets the needs of people in the community and that's a whole lot cheaper for us. At the end of the financial year, we said to people can you return any unspent money to us – we got over £200,000 returned to us. People are much more frugal with their resources than we would be."

The future of personalised commissioning

There are a number of future challenges that will shape the ways in which commissioning for personalisation develops. These include the current economic situation, a series of political changes following the 2010 General Election and a number of longer-term demographic, social and cultural changes. The future funding of social care – which will shape eligibility for state-funded personal budgets – has been a highly contentious issue, with the major parties divided on how to proceed. The independent commission set up by the Liberal–Conservative government is charged with examining a range of funding options in order to create 'an affordable and sustainable funding system for care and support, for all adults in England' (see http://carecommission.dh.gov.uk/). The future of personalisation in relation to health and social care is also likely to be contingent on the impact of the reorganisation of the NHS into general practitioner (GP) commissioning consortia, and the abolition of PCTs and strategic health authorities (DH, 2010).

Two possible scenarios can be envisaged. First, there is a possibility that the transformatory spirit of personalisation will be lost as it becomes routinised and mainstreamed. Certainly some of the initial creativity and support that has been possible looks hard to support on a mainstream basis. As one local authority support planner explained, "It is taking a long time to do a support plan ... I can do three or four at a time.... Social workers have caseloads of 50 to 60 older people. They haven't got time to do a support plan."

In the face of resource challenges, some interviewees raised concerns that the radical promise of personalisation would come to little: "In the first year [of having a personal budget] most people buy the same thing as before. The biggest risk in all this is that nothing will really change" (local authority social care manager). Although the numbers of people on personal budgets are rising, some people fear that this is a rebadging process, as 'care plans' are renamed 'support plans' without the transfer of choice and control to the service user that self-directed support envisages. As one director of adult social care said: "The question is, is it just a piece of paper saying you have got £100 but nothing has really changed?"

In contrast to this is the model of redevelopment set out by Duffy and others, in which personalisation is the trigger for a reworking of the whole post-1945 welfare settlement. Here the changes in social care cascade into a wider system change, in which everything from education to the tax and benefit system is reworked on a personalised basis (Glasby et al, 2010). The assumption is that a slow start will gradually escalate into systemic change, as 'tipping points' are reached, where sufficient levels of participation in new schemes lead to new patterns of contracting and disinvestment (OPM, 2008, p 38). A Demos report, looking at how people are likely to spend their social care budgets in the future, found some support for this, noting: 'There is some indication that the longer people have a personal budget, the more radical they will become in considering ways of spending their budget money' (Bartlett, 2009, p 27).

If personalisation is the basis for a welfare state in which payments to service users become the norm in a range of sectors, the impact on local authority commissioners is unclear. There is a scenario in which the state plays an active role in shaping and regulating markets, supporting users to be effective micro-commissioners through ensuring the supply of information and advocacy, and helping providers to deal with the demand risks of the new commissioning context. However, there is an alternative scenario of state withdrawal in which markets are left to reach equilibrium and individual budget holders use informal and third sector support to navigate the options available to them, bearing greater risk as the price of increased choice and control. It is as yet unclear which of these scenarios is supported by the current government and likely to be the basis of commissioning in the future.

Conclusion

Commissioning for personalisation constitutes a substantial shift in the models of commissioning that have been developing in local authorities. Issues for commissioners are likely to focus on certain nodal points: supporting individual users as micro-commissioners; stimulating and shaping local markets, what the Department of Health calls 'operational commissioning'; and then the broader issues of strategic commissioning, linked to integrated services and the management of risk and shrinking budgets.

Current practice in social care indicates that there is a range of problems currently being experienced as new models of commissioning emerge. These are focused on a lack of information, undeveloped services, poor integration between services, low levels of trust between local authorities, service users and providers, and a worsening financial context. It is as yet unclear whether these limitations will constrain the impact of personalisation within social care, or whether a critical mass of personal budget holders will find creative ways to build relationships and work around financial shortages.

The impact of personalisation to date has been felt most strongly in social care. However, pilots in children's services and healthcare indicate that a range of professionals must soon adjust to a new commissioning environment. Given the ambitious restructuring of the NHS envisaged by the Liberal–Conservative government, a whole new set of professionals based in GP consortia will be required to negotiate the terrain between individual, operational and strategic commissioning. It is difficult to read across from personal budgets in social care to personal health budgets given the different professional norms and user relationships that exist between social workers and GPs. It is clear only that for the NHS, as for social care, past commissioning models will be of limited use in understanding the future.

Further reading

- ACEVO (Association of Chief Executives of Voluntary Organisations) (2009) *Making it personal: a social market revolution – the interim report of the ACEVO Commission on Personalisation*, London: ACEVO.
- Carr, S. (2010) *Personalisation: a rough guide* (revised edition), London: Social Care Institute for Excellence.
- Department of Health (2008) *Commissioning for personalisation: a framework for local authority commissioners*, London: DH.
- Duffy, S. (2008) *Smart commissioning: exploring the impact of personalisation on commissioning*, Wythall: In Control.
- Glasby, J. and Littlechild, R. (2009) *Direct payments and personal budgets: putting personalisation into practice* (2nd edition), Bristol: The Policy Press.
- Needham, C. (2010) *Commissioning for personalisation: from the fringes to the mainstream*, London: CIPFA/Public Management and Policy Association.

- Needham, C. (2011) *Personalising public services: understanding the personalisation narrative*, Bristol: The Policy Press.

Useful websites

- Centre for Welfare Reform: www.centreforwelfarereform.org/
- In Control: www.in-control.org.uk/
- Office for Public Management: www.opm.co.uk/
- Social Care Institute for Excellence: www.scie.org.uk/
- Unison: www.unison.org.uk/localgov/personalisation.asp

Reflective exercises

1. If you were using adult social care services, would you want to receive a directly provided service or would you want the option of a personal budget? What sort of factors might influence your decision and what sort of information and support would you want before deciding?
2. If personal budgets are being rolled out across adult social care, what implications could they have in other areas of the welfare state?
3. How might commissioning in an era of personalisation differ from previous approaches?
4. In future, what sort of services would you want to commission en masse via a block contract and which might individuals want/be well placed to micro-commission themselves?

References

ACEVO (Association of Chief Executives of Voluntary Organisations) (2009) *Making it personal: a social market revolution – the interim report of the ACEVO Commission on Personalisation*, London: ACEVO.

ADASS (Association of Directors of Adult Social Services) (2009) *Personalisation and the law: implementing Putting People First in the current legal context*, London: ADASS.

Allen, K., Glasby, J. and Ham, C. (2009) *Integrating health and social care: a rapid review of lessons from evidence and experience*, Birmingham: Health Services Management Centre, University of Birmingham.

Audit Commission (2009) *Supporting People programme 2005-2009*, London: Audit Commission.

Bartlett, J. (2009) *At your service: navigating the future market in health and social care*, London: Demos.

Campbell, R. J., Robinson, W., Neelands, J., Hewston, R. and Mazzoli, L. (2007) 'Personalised learning: ambiguities in theory and practice', *British Journal of Educational Studies*, vol 55, no 2, pp 135-54.

Carr, S. (2010) *Personalisation: a rough guide* (revised edition), London: Social Care Institute for Excellence.

Concilium (2009) *Social enterprises working with prisons and probation services: a mapping exercise for National Offender Management Service*, London: Ministry of Justice/Cabinet Office.

Cowen, A. (2010) *Personalised transition: innovations in health, education and support*, Sheffield: Centre for Welfare Reform.

Crosby, N. (2010) *Personalisation: children, young people and families*, Wythall: In Control.

Cutler, T., Waine, B. and Brehony, K. (2007) 'A new epoch of individualization? Problems with the "personalization" of public sector services', *Public Administration*, vol 85, no 3, pp 847-55.

Darzi, A. (2007) *Our NHS, our future: NHS next stage review: interim report*, London: Department of Health.

Darzi, A. (2008) *High quality care for all: NHS next stage review: final report*, London: Department of Health.

DfES (Department for Education and Skills) (2007) *Aiming high for disabled children: better support for families*, London: HM Treasury/DfES.

DH (2006) *Our health, our care, our say: a new direction for community services*, London: DH.

DH (2008) *Commissioning for personalisation: a framework for local authority commissioners*, London: DH.

DH (2009a) *Personal health budgets: first steps*, London: DH.

DH (2009b) *Contracting for personalised outcomes: lessons from the emerging evidence*, London: DH.

DH (2010) *Equity and excellence: liberating the NHS*, London: TSO.

DH Care Networks (2009) *Personalisation*, www.dhcarenetworks.org.uk/IndependentLivingChoices/Housing/Topics/browse/Homelessness1/No_One_Left_Out/Personalisation/

Donnelly, L., Howie, M. and Leach, B. (2010) 'Councils pay for prostitutes for the disabled', *Daily Telegraph*, 14 August.

Dowson, S. and Greig, R. (2009) 'The emergence of the independent support broker role', *Journal of Integrated Care*, vol 17, no 4, pp 22-30.

Duffy, S. (2010) *The future of personalisation: implications for welfare reform*, Sheffield: Centre for Welfare Reform.

Duffy, S. and Fulton, K. (2009) *Should we ban brokerage?*, Sheffield: Centre for Welfare Reform/Paradigm.

Duffy, S., Waters, J. and Glasby, J. (2010) *Personalisation and the social care revolution: future options for the reform of public services*, Policy Paper 3, Birmingham: Health Services Management Centre, University of Birmingham.

DWP (Department for Work and Pensions) (2008) *No one written off: reforming welfare to reward responsibility*, London: TSO.

ECCA (English Community Care Association) (2010) *Personalising care: a route map to delivery for care providers*, London: ECCA.

Glasby, J., Duffy, S. and Needham, C. (2010) 'A Beveridge report for the twenty-first century? The implications of self-directed support for future welfare reform', paper presented to two-day think tank, Health Services Management Centre, University of Birmingham, June.

Glendinning, C., Challis, D., Fernandez, J., Jacobs, S., Jones, K., Knapp, M., Manthorpe, J., Moran, N., Netten, A., Stevens, M. and Wilberforce, M. (2008) *Evaluation of the individual budgets pilot programme*, York: Social Policy Research Unit.

Gove, M. (2010) *Written ministerial statement to Parliament*, 26 July.

HM Government (2007) *Putting People First: a shared vision and commitment to the transformation of adult social care*, London: HM Government.

HM Government (2010) *The coalition: our programme for government*, London: Cabinet Office.

Keohane, N. (2009) *People power: how can we personalise public services*, London: NLGN.

Leadbeater, C. (2004) *Personalisation through participation: a new script for public services*, London: Demos.

Leece, J. and Bornat, J. (eds) (2006) *Developments in direct payments*, Bristol: The Policy Press.

Mansell, J. (2010) *Raising our sights: services for adults with profound intellectual and multiple disabilities*, London: Department of Health.

Mansell, J. and Beadle-Brown, J. (2005) 'Person-centred planning and person-centred action: a critical perspective', in P. Cambridge and S. Carnaby (eds) *Person-centred planning and care management with people with learning disabilities*, London: Jessica Kingsley Publishers, pp 19-33.

Miliband, D. (2004) Speech to the North of England Education conference, January.

Needham, C. (2010) *Commissioning for personalization: from the fringes to the mainstream*, London: CIPFA/Public Management and Policy Association.

OPM (Office for Public Management) (2008) *Budget-holding lead professional pilots: final report*, London: OPM.

Poll, C. (2007) 'Co-production in supported housing: KeyRing living support networks and neighbourhood networks', in S. Hunter and P. Ritchie (eds) *Co-production and personalisation in social care changing relationships in the provision of social care*, London: Jessica Kingsley Publishers, pp 49-66.

Poll, C., Duffy, S., Hatton, C., Sanderson, H. and Routledge, M. (2006) *A report on In Control's first phase, 2003-2005*, London: In Control Publications.

SSAT (Specialist Schools and Academies Trust) (2010) *Personalisation briefing*, London: SSAT.

Taylor Knox, H. (2009) *Personalisation and individual budgets: challenge or opportunity?*, York: Housing Quality Network.

Tyson, A., Brewis, R., Crosby, N., Hatton, C., Stansfield, J., Tomlinson, C., Waters, J. and Wood, A. (2010) *A report on In Control's third phase: evaluation and learning 2008-2009*, London: In Control.

Part Three

Conclusion and next steps

TWELVE

Conclusion and next steps

Jon Glasby

Summary

This chapter sets out/explores:
- key themes from the book;
- implications for future policy and practice;
- implications for future research.

Since the early 1980s, the nature and delivery of public services such as health and social care have undergone a number of significant changes. One of the most important and far-reaching of these has arguably been the growing emphasis over time on the separation of commissioning and provision – sometimes into separate parts of the same public service organisation and sometimes into entirely separate organisational entities. Under the influence of broader political and economic trends, commissioning has therefore emerged as a core function and almost as a profession in its own right. However, these changes have not always been accompanied by the development of a sufficient infrastructure to give commissioners the confidence, skills and support they need to live up to the very rigorous demands of policy – and a book such as this is just one attempt to begin redressing this balance (albeit in a very small way).

Key themes

Writing from a range of different health, social care, local government and commercial perspectives, contributors to this book have identified a series of key themes as well as a number of outstanding issues and questions. Although these are too complex to reiterate in detail, this short conclusion seeks to draw together some of the overarching messages.

Implications for future policy and practice

- Although commissioning has often been the responsibility of 'managers', the advent of general practitioner (GP) commissioning means that the concepts explored in this book will be of increasing relevance to a range of health and social care practitioners and clinicians.

• There are many different types of commissioning, so local services need to be clear about which approach they are adopting and why (see Table 1.3 in Chapter One).

• Different agencies have different approaches to assessing the needs of their local populations (both technically and culturally). In an ideal world, there would be scope to learn from each other and to use mechanisms such as the joint strategic needs assessment as a means to understand jointly the health and social care needs of the local area.

• Priority setting seems to be undertaken differently in health and social care, with scope for additional joint work to help understand the rationale for this, the processes adopted and the outcomes achieved.

• Purchasing organisations are often political rather than rational in nature, and commissioning, contracting and procurement functions require attention to broader issues such as negotiation, power, relationship building, trust and understanding organisational behaviour.

• For all the debates that are under way about commissioning, policy tends to focus much less on the issue of *de*commissioning – and this seems a key gap in the current context.

• Too few commissioners seem to possess the skills and knowledge needed to assess the vulnerability/resilience of the services they are commissioning – and this seems a crucial development need in future.

• Despite ongoing emphasis on commissioning for quality and outcomes, prescriptive performance management arrangements can discourage innovation and creativity from providers.

• Health and social care face ongoing 'make-or-buy' decisions – and policy could be clearer about when it is best to deliver a service in-house and when commissioners should look externally.

• Public and patient engagement can be promoted for different reasons – and this influences the approach adopted and the definition of what success might look like. Being clear about underlying values and motives is therefore crucial.

• Despite ongoing policy commitment to 'joint commissioning', this should not be an end in itself – but simply a means to an end (of better services and better outcomes). Being clear about what joint commissioning is meant to achieve, for whom and how is therefore paramount.

• Chapter Eleven poses a clear policy challenge: 'Current practice in social care indicates that there is a range of problems currently being experienced as new models of commissioning emerge. These are focused on a lack of information, undeveloped services, poor integration between services, low levels of trust between local authorities, service users and providers, and a worsening financial context. It is as yet unclear whether these limitations will constrain the impact of personalisation within social care, or whether a critical mass of personal budget holders will find creative ways to build relationships and work around financial shortages.'

Implications for future research

- With a new government (2010-) and in an era of resource constraints, there are key questions as to whether strategic commissioning can deliver better outcomes, achieve greater value for money and meet rising public expectations at the same time (and whether commissioning is any better at this than other possible approaches). The emphasis placed on GP commissioning in particular is an important area for future research, and this will need careful evaluation as it develops.

- Needs assessment and priority setting are often portrayed as technical exercises, yet involve significant value judgements and raise issues around accountability and leadership. Additional research could usefully compare and contrast these different approaches – and the role of citizens and the public may be a particularly important area for further work.

- Research into decision making and priority setting could also usefully focus on issues of implementation and legitimacy in order to understand *how* commissioners' decisions are embedded and enacted locally (or not).

- There is a series of unanswered questions about the impact of payment mechanisms such as payment by results and Commissioning for Quality and Innovation (CQUIN) on costs, value for money, outcomes and local relationships. Although there has been more of a market in social care than in health (until recently), we still know less about the impact of commissioning in social care than we do in health.

- When evaluating the decommissioning of health and social services, there is scope to draw on the Maslin Multi-Dimensional Matrix from Chapters Five to Six and on the six perspectives from Chapter Five to structure the research.

- Chapter Six poses a direct question: 'Why is it that some providers fail to adapt to a changing environment? In particular, what dimensions or factors contribute to this lack of resilience and inability to manage change?'

- We may need to know more about what kind of outcomes service users want their health and social care services to be achieving on their behalf and how this might differ from the views of service providers, commissioners and policy makers.

- When and under what circumstances should health and social care organisations deliver services in-house and when should they commission services from others – and what impact might these different approaches have?

- More research is needed into whether/how public and patient engagement influences services and subsequent outcomes.

- In 1998, Glendinning et al (1998, p 124) asked: 'Which model of joint commissioning delivers most gains for patients? How easy is it for them to find out about services? Are services better coordinated? To what extent are patients' preferences taken into account? What are the consequences for equity and citizenship?' More than a decade later, these questions remain unanswered and are arguably even more important now than they were then.

- In future, research could help us to understand what is best commissioned by the individual, what needs commissioning at an operational level and what should be commissioned at a strategic level.

Overall, the strategic commissioning agenda has emerged in different ways in different departments/areas, with a resulting lack of clarity about key terms, rationales and intended outcomes. Joined-up development and educational opportunities may be one way forward in the absence of joined-up policy. Above all, we still know relatively little about the impact of strategic commissioning compared to other, more traditional ways of organising. Perhaps one option would be to conduct research into a series of local case studies, each using different ways of delivering services, and/or to make use of the natural experiments emerging in different parts of the United Kingdom in an era of devolution. Either way, strategic commissioning – and the skills and knowledge that underpin it – seems here to stay – and we hope that this book has helped to start to make sense of a complex and rapidly evolving agenda.

Reflective exercises

1. This chapter has summarised some of the key themes in the book as a whole and identified a series of outstanding questions for research, policy and practice. Having read the different contributions in this edited textbook, what are the key themes and recommendations you will take away?
2. If you were the Secretary of State responsible for new policy in this area, what would you do in response to these issues?
3. If you were a researcher interested in public service commissioning, what research questions would you ask and be keen to research?
4. If you were reading a book on this topic 10 years from now, what differences in topic and approach would you expect to see?

Reference

Glendinning, C., Rummery, K. and Clarke, R. (1998) 'From collaboration to commissioning: developing relationships between primary health and social services', *British Medical Journal*, vol 323, pp 122-5.

Index